Activity
Analysis
Handbook
Second Edition

Activity
Analysis
Handbook

Second Edition

Nancy K. Lamport, MS, OTR
Assistant Professor of Occupational Therapy

Margaret S. Coffey, MA, COTA, ROH
former Lecturer of Occupational Therapy

Gayle I. Hersch, PhD, OTR
Clinical Assistant Professor of Occupational Therapy

SLACK Incorporated, 6900 Grove Road, Thorofare, NJ 08086-9447

Printed in the United States of America

Library of Congress Catalog Card Number: 92-60370

ISBN 1-55642-215-6

Published by: SLACK Incorporated
               6900 Grove Road
               Thorofare, NJ 08086-9447

Last digit is print number: 10   9   8   7   6   5   4   3   2

Contents

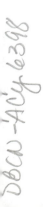

Appendices

Acknowledgments

The authors continue to see the *Activity Analysis Handbook* as an expanding rather than a definitive work. The authors gratefully acknowledge the many contributors to this lengthy endeavor. Erna Simek, MS, OTR, FAOTA, founder of the Occupational Therapy Assistants Program at Indiana University, first suggested the use of Uniform Terminology as the framework for activity analysis. Susan Meyers, EdD, OTR developed the first computer program for the activity analysis and patient-activity correlation. Medical Illustrations of Indiana University provided the graphics. Patricia Gerlach manned the word processor and assisted with layout in the First Edition. Roberta Fehrman patiently assisted with the Second Edition.

A special tribute goes to the baccalaureate and associate degree students of the Department of Occupational Therapy, School of Allied Health Sciences, Indiana University School of Medicine. Their examples of completed student assignments are the heart of the handbook. Without their questions, problem-solving skills, patience, and perseverance, this manual would not have been possible. And so, to them and to all the students and faculty who will contribute to this growing base of knowledge, we dedicate this Second Edition.

Nancy K. Lamport, MS, OTR
Margaret S. Coffey, MA, COTA, ROH
Gayle I. Hersch, PhD, OTR

About the Authors

Nancy K. Lamport, MS, OTR

Ms. Lamport is Assistant Professor of Occupational Therapy. Her teaching responsibilities are in the areas of activity analysis, daily life skills, and media. Her area of special interest is in home and community accessibility. She is affiliated with the Department of Occupational Therapy, School of Allied Health Sciences, Indiana University School of Medicine, Indianapolis, Indiana.

Margaret S. Coffey, MA, COTA, ROH

Ms. Coffey is a former Lecturer of Occupational Therapy in the Associate Degree and Baccalaureate Programs. Her teaching responsibilities included group activities and media. She currently practices in long-term care facilities.

Gayle I. Hersch, PhD, OTR

Ms. Hersch is a Clinical Assistant Professor of Occupational Therapy with teaching responsibilities in the areas of human development, media and research. She is also the fieldwork coordinator for the OT program. Her area of expertise is gerontology. She is affiliated with the Department of Occupational Therapy, School of Allied Health Sciences, Indiana University School of Medicine, Indianapolis, Indiana.

Preface

The evolution of the First Edition of the *Activity Analysis Handbook* began in 1983. A faculty ad hoc committee was charged with the development of a consistent method for teaching the concepts of activity analysis to baccalaureate and associate degree students. While the subject of activity analysis was valued by the faculty, there was no ownership or consistency in the presentation of the material.

This charge generated several years of research, an ongoing review of activity analysis forms currently in use, and finally, the development of the activity analysis form as it is presented in the First Edition. Concurrently, with the development of the activity analysis structure, the concepts of activity awareness and activity identification also needed attention in the teaching of activity analysis and were incorporated into the handbook format. Finally, the patient-activity correlation was developed as the culminating agent for the other three concepts. Uniform Terminology for Reporting Occupational Therapy Services (UTS) provided the foundation for the developing process.

A revision of the *Activity Analysis Handbook* was initiated due to classroom experiences coupled with the Second Edition of Uniform Terminology. In this revised handbook both editions of Uniform Terminology appear. The charts and forms which are based on the first Uniform Terminology are retained in their original format. Revisions to these, according to Uniform Terminology II, can be found in Appendix C.

In the classroom, the students observed that they needed more consistency and less variety in the activities they applied to the forms. Therefore, in this Second Edition, the same activity is processed through all four of the forms. To expand the students' thinking, Chapter 3 highlights student examples of completed activity analysis and patient-activity correlation. This section was developed to demonstrate some of the many ways that activity can be therapeutically applied to a variety of patients or clients and in a variety of settings. The course instructors developed new teaching strategies and some of these have been incorporated in the expanded section devoted to learning resources. The computer section found in the First Edition has been deleted. Instructors found that students used their own familiar software to complete their assignments successfully. The authors hope that these revisions are indicative of the continuing growth of this body of knowledge.

Introduction

Activity Analysis: An Interactive Process

The philosophical base of occupational therapy rests upon purposeful activity. Knowledge and a thorough understanding of purposeful activity become crucial to the student of occupational therapy. Underlying this understanding is a particular way of thinking about activity as a means of helping people achieve, maintain or return to productive lives.

This text provides the occupational therapy student with a method for developing the critical thinking skills required to identify, analyze and adapt activities that are potentially useful as treatment modalities in the practice of occupational therapy. This method imparts to the student the thought processes involved in choosing activities for use in treatment and the correlation of these activities with specific patient needs. A student's personal experience in performing activities becomes the means for understanding the inherent nature and therapeutic benefits of purposeful activity.

The basic approach of this book is twofold. First, purposeful activity should be examined as it is normally performed. Second, specific activities or components of an activity will correlate with a given patient's treatment needs through precise treatment implications. Four forms are used to reflect this dual approach and to provide the opportunity to develop a particular thought process with regard to the use of purposeful activity in occupational therapy. This thought process is commonly called "activity analysis." Building an understanding of what is involved in activity, and how using that activity with a patient makes a difference, is the major thrust of this book.

The forms should be used in a sequential manner in order to link the value of activity with the therapeutic use of activity in occupational therapy. As this mode of thinking develops, the analysis of activity becomes a conscious thought process with all activities used in treatment. The student moves from a basic understanding of activity to the practice of activity analysis and finally to an evaluation of an activity's major contributions in clinical practice. All major facets of an activity are explored, and skills needed to engage in an activity are identified. Problem-solving is facilitated by addressing the performance of an activity in which the patient's skills are weak or absent. The relationship between the health of the individual and the performance of the activity are integrated.

In this text, UTS becomes the basis for recording the component parts of an activity and for documenting the outcome of the use of activity in treatment. All treatment outcomes resulting from occupational therapy intervention are observable, measurable and subject to documentation. With the revision of Uniform Terminology, changes have been made in the occupational performance charts (Appendix C). However, the main headings and subdivisions used in the examples and worksheets found in the text adhere to the first UTS.

The application of activity analysis is seen as a sequencing process, one step building upon another, integrating a growing knowledge about common problems and conditions seen in occupational therapy with a knowledge of activity. The study of activity and the appreciation of activity as the medium of occupational therapy is a guiding concept throughout this text. The ability to document the use and importance of purposeful activity in treatment is a goal for every occupational therapy student.

Objectives

Upon completion of the use of this handbook, the learner should be able to:

- understand the inherent qualities found in purposeful activities and the effect of engaging in such activities on the health of the individual.

- express activities in descriptive terms, separating out actions used to perform the activity in task sequence.

- analyze an activity in terms of the component skills required to perform it and the occupational performance areas involved in doing so.

- list the physical and environmental requirements for performing an activity, including precautions or contraindications, and acceptable criteria to determine successful completion of the activity.

- define and apply the principles of activity analysis in the practice of occupational therapy through preparing analyses of activities as they are normally performed.

- formulate alternative means of performing the activity in an acceptable manner through adaptation or modification of equipment, environment or the activity.

- practice problem-solving skills in selecting activities to meet specific needs of a patient receiving occupational therapy services.

- propose treatment goals for therapy based on the use of an activity with a given patient applicable to the performance ares of work, play and daily living skills.

- apply Uniform Terminology to describe, analyze and document the use of activities in the practice of occupational therapy.

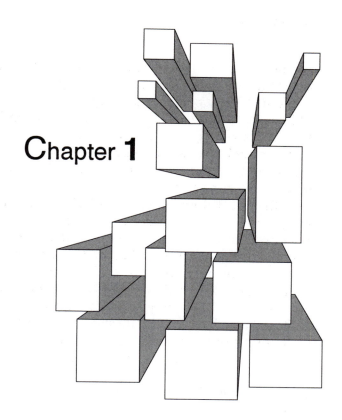

Chapter 1

EXAMINING THE PROCESS

Historical Perspective of Activity

"The proper use of time in some helpful and gratifying activity appeared. . . a fundamental issue in the treatment of any. . .patient" (Meyer, 1922, p. 1).

The heritage of activity in the profession of occupational therapy can be traced to the late 1800s. During that time, Adolph Meyer recognized the value of work and occupation to his neuropsychiatric patients. The above quote, taken from a paper presented at the fifth Annual Meeting of the National Society for the Promotion of Occupational Therapy (now the American Occupational Therapy Association) in October 1921, reflects Meyer's personal commitment to the promotion of activity in the psychosocial and physical treatment of patients. He described this treatment method as the "new scheme." In his words, therapeutic work "was a pleasure in achievement, a real pleasure in the use and activity of one's hands and muscles and a happy appreciation of time" (Meyer, 1921, p. 3). Sprinkled throughout this historical document are words such as performance, energy-transformers, interest, adaptation and integration, words familiar to any contemporary occupational therapist.

Wilma West, a prominent occupational therapist, reiterated the belief that activity is the philosophical base of occupational therapy and identified several sources in the professional literature (West, 1984). Especially noteworthy is Mary Reilly's hypothesis "that man, through the use of his hands, as they are energized by mind and will, can influence the state of his own health" (Reilly, 1962, p. 8). This is reminiscent of Meyer's "new scheme" (Figure 1-1).

With such theoretical statements, however, comes the burden of proof. Health practice in general, and occupational therapy in particular, is being held accountable for its treatment and techniques. Documentation of treatment in clear and succinct terms is essential for occupational therapy to thrive in today's health market.

This dichotomy may cause the student and therapist to ask the following questions:

How, then, does activity energize the cognitive skills of the mind?

How, then, does activity motivate the functional being?

How, then, does activity influence one's health?

These are provocative questions that need substantive answers. History has challenged the occupational therapy profession to act responsibly to insure successful outcomes (Figure 1-2). One way is by analyzing activity in all of its distinct parts, thereby establishing justification for its use in treatment and its contribution to the health of the individual.

Purposeful Activity

As the student explores the historical roots of our profession, a number of definitions of occupational therapy will be identified. Some of the definitions are lengthy, some are more succinct. All of them reflect a sincere attempt to explain and interpret the purpose and scope of occupational therapy. The thoughtful student will begin to realize that regardless of the period of time in which a definition was formed, there is a common thread which is: activity, used in a purposeful way, can facilitate a positive change in a person's level of function.

The following definition of occupational therapy was adopted in 1986 by the Representative Assembly of the American Occupational Therapy Association.

Occupational therapy is the therapeutic use of self-care, work, and play activities to increase independent function, enhance development and prevent disability. It may include adaptation of task or environment to achieve maximum independence and to enhance quality of life.

If purposeful activity is the key concept in occupational therapy, then what is an activity and how does the therapist use it? Trombly describes activity as "anything that requires mental processing of data, physical manipulation of objects, or direct movement" (Trombly, 1983, p. 242).

In 1982 the Representative Assembly of the American Occupational Therapy Association officially adopted the position paper that sets forth the use of purposeful activity as a legitimate tool used by occupational therapists to evaluate, facilitate, restore, and maintain function (see *Purposeful Activities: A Position Paper*, Appendix A).

The "purpose" in purposeful activity is to bring forth a calculated response from the patient to the activity that addresses his treatment goals. Depending upon therapy goals,

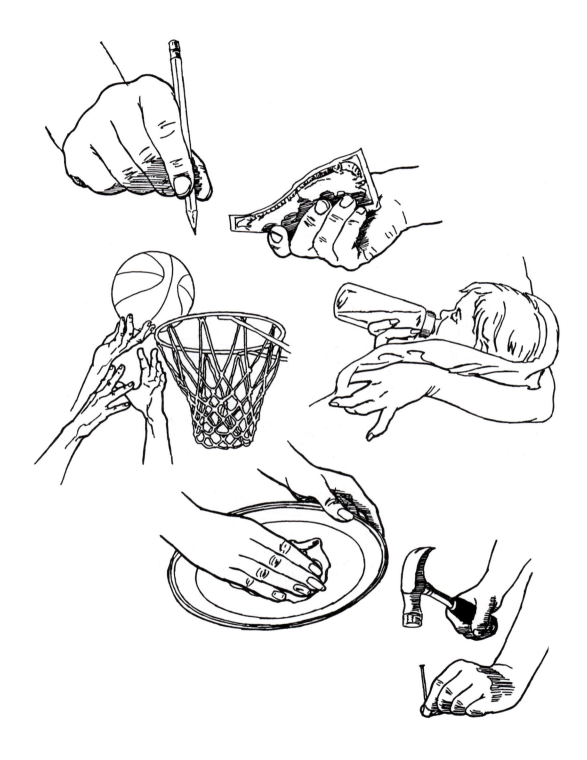

Figure 1-1.   *"Man, through the use of his hands, as they are energized by mind and will,*
can influence the state of his own health."

M. Reilly — 1962

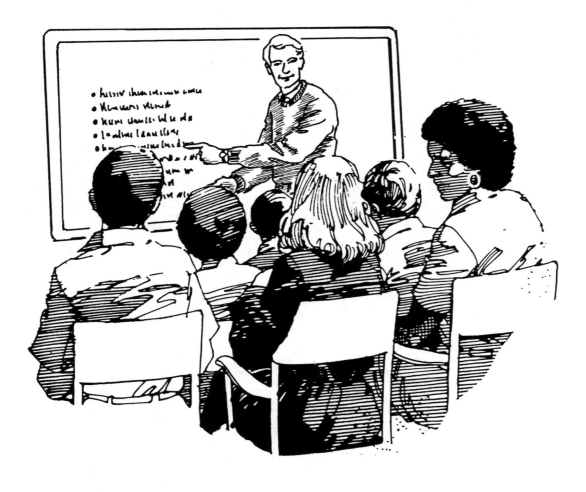

Figure 1-2.   *"Our educators must begin to base the curricula on our value system of occupation and the occupational process, and on the science of occupation and the art of purposefulness."*
E. Gilfoyle — 1984

the performance of the activity can provide the means to increase strength, encourage social interaction, decrease anxiety, or stimulate cognitive function. Activities can be graded, sequenced or monitored; they can be facilitative, protective or adaptive. The key point is that as the patient is involved in the activity, he is working toward increased function.

Occupational Performance and the Uniform Terminology System

The goal of occupational therapy is functional independence in the three areas of occupational performance: physical and psychosocial daily living skills, work and play/leisure. The therapist communicates goals of therapy, patient progress and other official documentation through the language of the Uniform Terminology System (UTS). With this system, the occupational therapist or an occupational therapy assistant can systematically formulate and realistically communicate potential and attainable results of occupational therapy (see Appendix B for the complete first edition of Uniform Terminology for Reporting Occupational Therapy Services and Appendix C for the Second Edition).

With the acceptance of the UTS, adopted by the Representative Assembly of the American Occupational Therapy Association in March 1981, the profession assumed a universal method of documentation applicable to all areas of occupational performance. UTS is applicable to note writing as well as to computer use in charting, reimbursement and research. With a uniform approach, therapists can communicate readily with each other, with third-party payers and with other professionals in a manner that will greatly reduce communication discrepancies due to subjective interpretation.

The Occupational Performance Chart

The occupational performance chart is a diagrammatical representation of the UTS, which allows the reader to visualize the totality of treatment with all its implicit components. The three-page representation (see Figures 1-3, 1-4, 1-5) depicts treatment as sequential and interactive. Performance categories are segmented into workable pieces, yet come together to form a holistic picture of treatment. The occupational performance chart (see Figure 1-3) provides the five major headings for the succeeding segments. These major headings are:

- Independent Living/Daily Living Skills

- Occupational Performance Components

- Occupational Performance Modification

- Life-Space Influences

- Independent Function

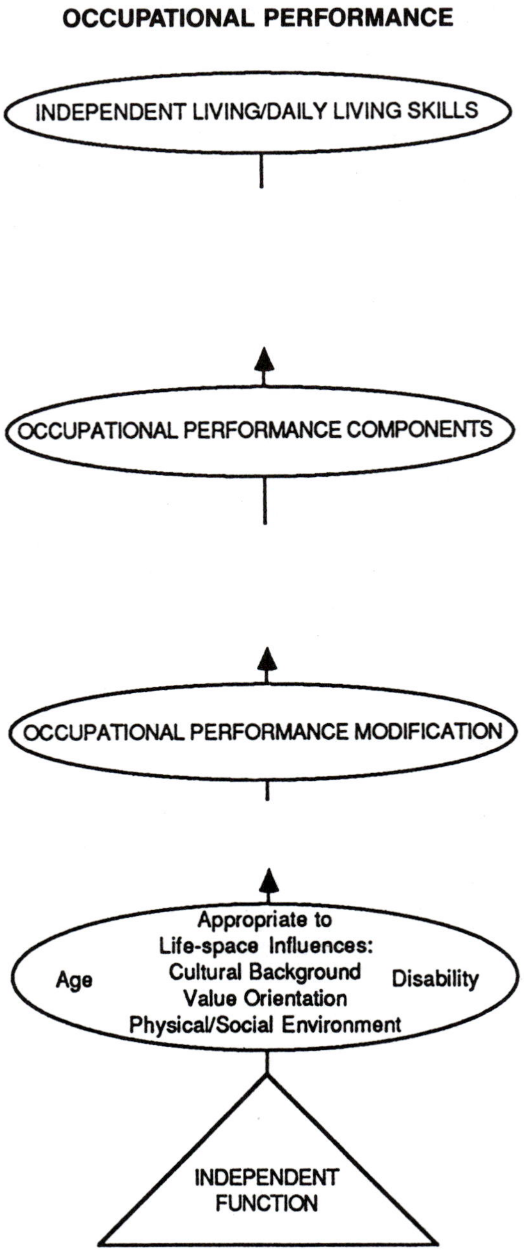

OCCUPATIONAL PERFORMANCE

INDEPENDENT LIVING/DAILY LIVING SKILLS

OCCUPATIONAL PERFORMANCE COMPONENTS

OCCUPATIONAL PERFORMANCE MODIFICATION

Appropriate to
Life-space Influences:
Age   Cultural Background   Disability
Value Orientation
Physical/Social Environment

INDEPENDENT
FUNCTION

Figure 1-3.

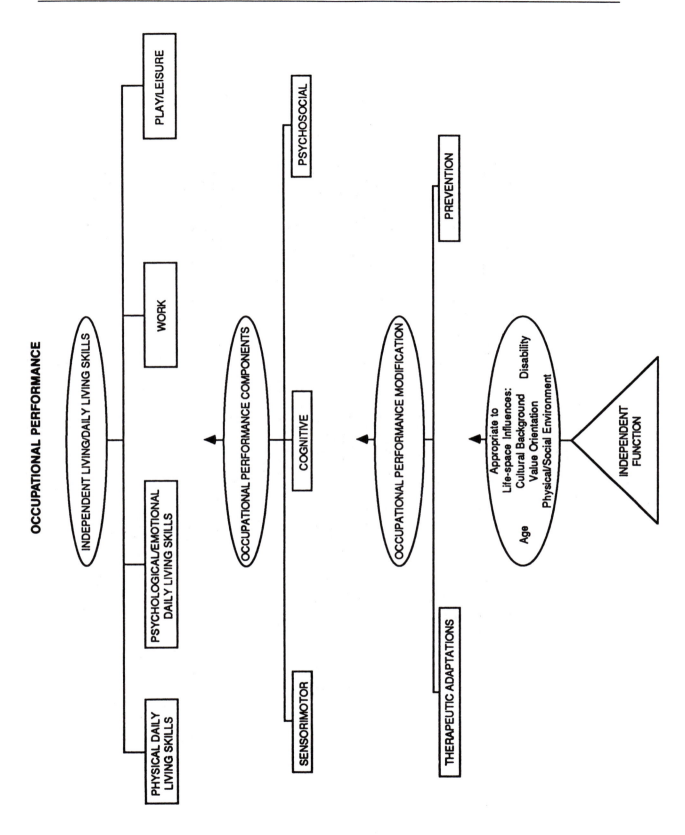

Figure 1-4.

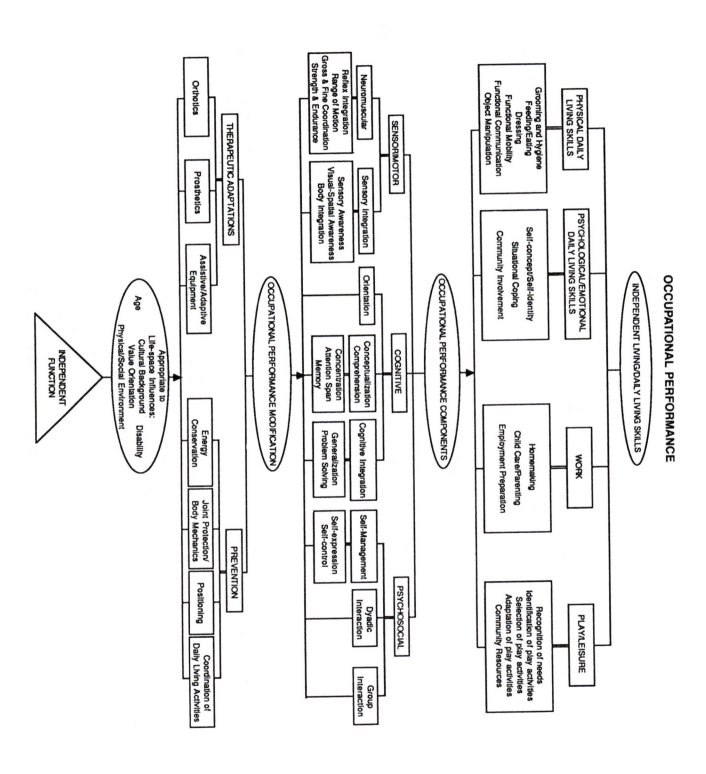

Figure 1-5.

Figure 1-4 inserts the major categories under each of the five headings, Figure 1-5 adds the tertiary row of UTS descriptions for each of the above categories. In this way, one segment of the document can be studied before proceeding to the next segment and before adding more details.

For example, the occupational performance area of physical daily living skills consists of five subareas: grooming and hygiene, feeding/eating, dressing, functional mobility, functional communication, and object manipulation. In addition, the sub-area of dressing may be differentiated into three patient performance components: sensorimotor, cognitive, and psychosocial. Within each of these components, additional factors may be considered, eg, range of motion, attention span, and self-management. By analyzing the normal skills inherent in each of these components, the therapist can make comparisons and determine a patient's level of function. If there are functional deficits, performance modifications can be made. Treatment may also include a therapeutic adaptation such as an assistive device or may incorporate a prevention technique such as positioning.

The ultimate goal is the independent functioning of the individual with consideration of the patient's age and disability, as well as life span influences that include cultural background, value orientation and physical social environment.

The diagram is a composite of treatment outcomes allowing for a kaleidoscope of variation. Understanding that each patient is an individual requiring a unique treatment plan, the occupational therapist or occupational therapy assistant can formulate an effective treatment regimen.

Rationale for the Activity Analysis Process

A key to treatment in occupational therapy is the careful identification of skills required for a prescribed activity as well as a thorough understanding of activity. The patient takes an active role in the treatment process by being involved in the choice of activities used; however, it is the therapist's professional judgment and application of the purposeful activities selected that determine the therapeutic effectiveness of the activity. A therapist's skill at analyzing activities is critical. Activity analysis is a problem-solving strategy that will:

- provide the therapist with a thorough understanding of the activity and assure a knowledge base for the instruction of the activity through directions, simplification or adaptation.

- contribute facts to the therapist regarding equipment, supplies and materials, cost, time, space and staff involvement required to perform the activity.

- generate knowledge for the therapist to judge the use of the activity regarding answers to the questions for whom, when, where, why and under what circumstances the activity would be therapeutic.

- equip the therapist with a justification for using the activity with patients by detailing the therapeutic benefits of the activity as defined by the analysis.

- supply information to the therapist that can be used to document patient progress in skills and abilities, levels of achievement, areas of difficulty, and reference points for treatment intervention.

There is no universal method for completing an activity analysis. Often the analysis is dependent upon the therapist's area of expertise, frame of reference, or personal preference. The following method is one approach to activity analysis that provides a format to develop the conscious thought processes for analyzing activities. It is a mechanism that provides organization for the many, many factors that impact treatment. In this approach there are no right or wrong answers, only a framework for reasoning.

Overview of the Activity Analysis Process

An occupational therapist focuses on an activity from two specific directions—as it is normally performed and as it is performed by the patient. Sometimes the normal performance and the patient's performance are similar. In occupational therapy, activity more often requires evaluation and restructuring to place it within the patient's range of ability. Lifespace influences and a holistic understanding of the patient determine the final choice of the activity.

To provide a knowledge of all these aspects of activity and to establish a structure for learning, four forms are presented in this text. These forms should be used in the sequence in which they are presented until the student feels competent following the directions and integrating the information provided by their use. The forms may then be used out of sequence to explore new activities or to approach a different understanding of familiar activities for potential use in occupational therapy. One copy of each form is included in the text and is followed by a completed student example. A set of blank forms for classroom use appears in Appendix D.

The Activity Awareness Form

The first form allows an activity to be viewed subconsciously and highlights the student's personal response to a specific activity. The physical, psychosocial and cognitive aspects of the activity are superficially identified.

The Action Identification Form

The second form provides a more direct approach to the composition of the activity and separates its major sequential steps. A broader scope of the ways it may be accomplished is recognized.

The Activity Analysis Form

The third form requires an intense examination of the occupational performance components of the activity. Sensorimotor, psychosocial and cognitive aspects of the activity are specifically identified and supported through the use of the UTS. Standard activity requirements and projected treatment implications are also recorded.

The Patient-Activity Correlation

The fourth form addresses the patient's treatment needs and the application of the activity as treatment. The form requires long- and short-term goals, identifies the activity of choice, and documents its use as a treatment modality using UTS. Since therapy results, and not the activity used, are the basis for documentation, the use of UTS provides a ready vehicle for the recording of treatment outcomes in concise, professional terms.

Occupational therapists learn to use activity as a therapeutic modality. The student begins by becoming aware of the many different activities and their inherent nature. Activities are then broken down into individual steps to identify their specific actions. Next, the value of an activity becomes magnified by analyzing the skills required to perform it. Finally, the patient's needs are assessed and an activity is correlated to address these needs. Throughout this process, the impact of life space, cultural background, value orientation, age, disability, and environmental influences is considered. This approach to activity analysis can be applied to any activity used in occupational therapy and is applicable to a variety of treatment settings.

References

American Occupational Therapy Association. (1979). *Uniform Terminology for Reporting Occupational Therapy Services.* Rockville, MD: AOTA.

Gilfoyle, E.M. (1984). Eleanor Clark Slagle Lectureship, 1984: Transformation of a profession. *The American Journal of Occupational Therapy, 38,* 575-584.

Meyer, A. (1922). The philosophy of occupational therapy. *Archives of Occupational Therapy, 1,* 1-10.

Reilly, M. (1962). Eleanor Clark Slagle Lectureship, Occupational therapy can be one of the great ideas of 20th century medicine. *The American Journal of Occupational Therapy, 16,* 1-9.

Trombly, C.A. (Ed). (1983). *Occupational Therapy for Physical Dysfunction.* 2nd edition.Baltimore: Williams & Wilkins.

West, W.A. (1984). A reaffirmed philosophy and practice of occupational therapy for the 1980s. *The American Journal of Occupational Therapy, 38,* 15-23.

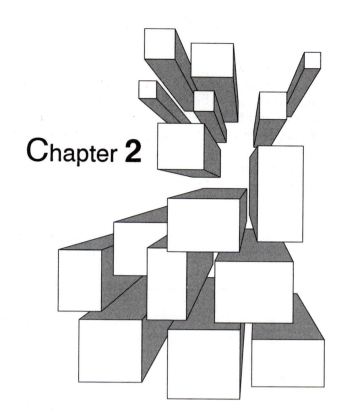

Chapter 2

EXPERIENCING THE PROCESS

This chapter presents, describes and explains the four types of activity analysis forms used in this book. Included are blank forms on which the student can practice activity analysis skills, as well as completed student examples. Blank versions of these forms, provided for classroom and clinical use, can be found in Appendix D.

Isolating the Activity

The Activity Awareness Form

Rationale

Understanding the inherent qualities of the activity provides a foundation for further analysis and defines therapeutic implications as treatment modalities. The intent of this form is to tap into the student's stream of consciousness. While doing an activity, the student is unaware of having any purpose other than what is apparent, i.e., opening a can or sanding wood for a project. It is only upon directed reflection that the student becomes conscious of more occurring than just "doing" the activity.

Objectives

Completing the Activity Awareness Form following the performance of an activity will help the student become more conscious of the hidden facets of the activity as it is usually performed by a healthy individual. An activity may be selected by the student or assigned by an instructor. Any simple activity is appropriate.

Directions

To complete the sample form, the student should choose and complete a simple activity, and:

- recall the thoughts and feelings spontaneously evoked by the activity. These may include memories, desires, hopes, and current concerns.

- recognize the general physical requirements of the activity.

- express the cognitive, physical or emotional stimulation the student experienced while doing the activity.

- detect the ongoing effect of an activity after its performance is completed.

- identify a personal response to the activity.

Form 2-1 is an example of a blank Activity Awareness form.

Form 2-2 is an example of a completed Activity Awareness form. The Activity Awareness form for completing the assignment is found in Appendix D (Student Worksheets).

Form 2-1.
ACTIVITY AWARENESS FORM

Student: _____ Date: _____
Activity: _____
Course: _____

Directions: Reflecting on the activity just performed, complete the following sentences with the first thoughts that come to mind.

1. During this activity I was thinking about. . .

2. While doing this activity I felt like. . .

3. In doing this activity, the parts of my body I remember using were. . .

4. To do this activity I need to. . .(mentally, emotionally, physically)

5. When I do this activity again I will. . .

6. From doing this activity I became aware of. . .

Form 2-2.
ACTIVITY AWARENESS FORM

Student: _Example_ _____ Date: _____
Activity: _Making a telephone call_ _____
Course: _____

Directions: Reflecting on the activity just performed, complete the following sentences with the first thoughts that come to mind.

1. During this activity I was thinking about. . .
   All the things I need to get done today and hoping the person was at home so that I could give her a message she needed to have before leaving her home.

2. While doing this activity I felt. . .
   Relieved when my friend answered the phone and I was able to talk to her.

3. In doing this activity, the parts of my body I remember using were. . .
   My leg while standing by the phone, my shoulder holding the phone against my ear, writing with my hand while she talked.

4. To do this activity, I needed to. . .
   Remember her phone number, dial accurately, listen for the phone to ring, wait for my friend to respond, and then relay the information needed.

5. When I do this activity again, I will. . .
   Sit down after dialing the wall phone and have my list in front of me to check off items as I complete them.

6. From doing this act, I became aware of. . .
   How anxious I was to convey the message and complete this job on my list.

Identifying the Components

The Action Identification Form

Rationale

Activities are more than they appear to be. They tap into a variety of skills and functions as they are performed. The activity as a treatment modality requires the student to distinguish the specific components of an activity from its general appearance and to develop the ability to describe these components in precise, objective terms (See Figures 2-1, 2-2).

Objectives

Action identification will move the student from a general perception of how the activity is performed to an identification of the specific actions taken in performing the activity. Upon completion of the Action Identification Form, the student should be able to:

- name an activity in descriptive terms.

- identify and separate the actions taken to perform the activity.

- describe the actions in a "Do-What-How" sentence format using a verb, noun and adverb. (T.A.S.K., A.C.T., 1979)

- observe similarities and differences in the way the same activity is performed by different people and at different times.

Directions

The student will choose one of the activities listed below, then record the major steps required to perform this activity (within ten or fewer steps) in the left-hand column of the Action Identification Form (Form 2-3). The student will use the "Do-What-How" format.

- writing a note

- tying a shoe

- removing a book from a bookbag

- drinking from a glass

- brushing teeth

- making a phone call

The student will observe someone else performing the same activity and record the observations in the second column of the Action Identification Form, noting similarities and differences.

As this form is completed, it is important to note that the significance of the direction (do) and the action (what) are probably more obvious than the descriptor (how). However, the descriptor identifies the quality of the action which is required or observed, as illustrated in the following examples:

- sit down slowly (a direction)

- the patient approached the task hesitantly (an observation)

Form 2-3 is an example of a blank Action Identification Form.

Form 2-4 is an example of a completed Action Identification Form. The Action Identification form for completing the assignment is found in Appendix D (Student Worksheets).

Form 2-3.
ACTION IDENTIFICATION FORM

Directions: Select an activity and list the major actions (in sequence) required for you to perform this activity *in ten or less steps* . Repeat the exercise after observing someone else perform the same activity. Use the "Do-What-How" format.

Student: _____ Date: _____

Activity selected: _____

Course: _____

Observation of Self	Observation of Another

Form 2-4.
ACTION IDENTIFICATION FORM

Directions: Select an activity and list the major actions (in sequence) required for you to perform this activity *in ten or less steps* . Repeat the exercise after observing someone else perform the same activity. Use the "Do-What-How" format.

Student: *Example* _____ Date: _____

Activity selected: *Making a phone call* _____

Course: _____

Observation of Self	Observation of Another
1. Open phone book slowly.	1. Find phone number carefully.
2. Find number carefully.	2. Pick up receiver firmly.
3. Lift up receiver gently.	3. Listen for dial tone carefully.
4. Listen for dial tone carefully.	4. Push correct numbers firmly.
5. Push buttons slowly.	5. Listen to ringing carefully.
6. Listen to other phone ring quietly.	6. Talk to person that answers respectfully.
7. Wait for response patiently.	7. Cease conversation courteously.
8. Say "hello" slowly.	8. Hang up receiver firmly.
9. Close conversation courteously.	
10. Put receiver down gently.	

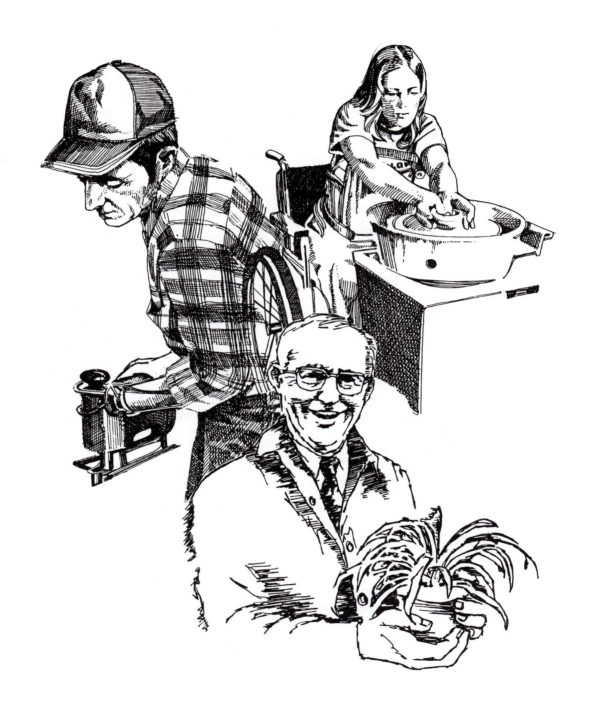

Figure 2-1. *"Activity is the medium of occupational therapy."*
C.A. Trombly — 1983

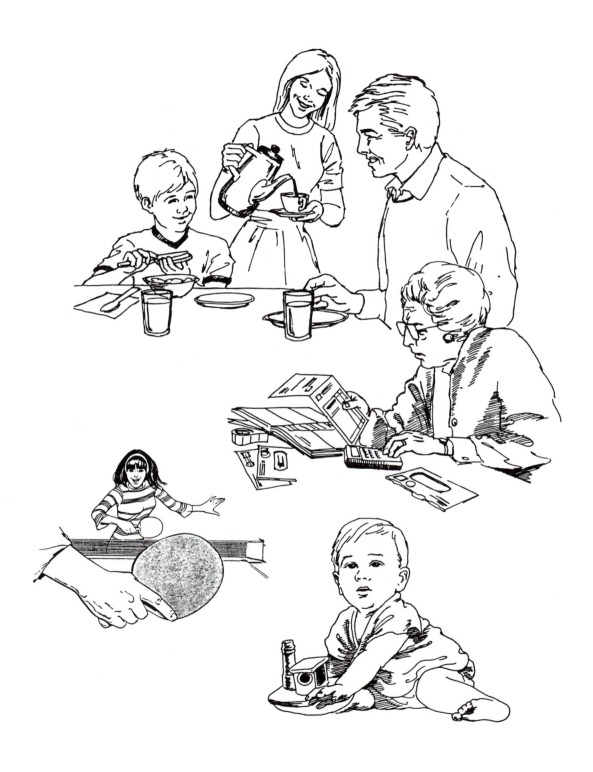

Figure 2-2.

"Anything that requires mental processing of data, physical manipulation of objects or directed movement may be considered an activity."

C.A. Trombly — 1983

Magnifying the Skills

The Activity Analysis Form

Rationale

According to Rogers (1984), to use occupation or purposeful activity effectively in treatment, the occupational therapist needs to have an in-depth understanding of the health-enhancing nature of occupation. This understanding does not come through memorization or demonstration. It evolves from knowing about normal occupational function, ineffective performance in occupational function, and the therapeutic properties of occupation. How does this conceptual formation occur? It involves a step-by-step dissection to uncover the obvious and to discover the meaning of the activity under consideration.

Part I - Activity Summary   The activity is identified and briefly described. Information regarding the equipment, supplies, costs, time requirements, utilization of space and staff involvement required to perform the activity are noted. Precautions, contraindications, age and educational requirements, as well as sexual and cultural relevance, are addressed. Acceptable criteria for a completed activity are determined.

Part II - Occupational Performance Components   The components of an occupation or purposeful activity are closely examined. Three aspects of the self emerge: the doing self (the physical or sensorimotor components), the thinking self (the cognitive components), and the feeling self (the socio-emotional aspects of the activity) (Crepeau, 1986). Analyzing the activity according to these factors facilitates the understanding of occupation. Conceptualization of purposeful activity, in all its dimensions, encourages the student to appreciate the holistic value of the task.

Part III - Occupational Performance   An activity can be applicable to one or more of the three major areas of occupational performance (daily living skills, work, and play/leisure).

Part IV - Occupational Performance Modifications   Modifications, adaptations, and/or preventative measures that may be required for the activity to become a therapeutic modality are considered.

Objectives

Upon completion of the Activity Analysis Form, the student should be able to:

- describe the supplies, equipment, and environmental requirements needed in doing the activity.

- identify the task sequence and acceptable criteria for completion of the activity.

- indicate precautions, contraindications, and any other special considerations associated with the performance of the activity.

- describe and analyze activities using UTS.

- examine the sensorimotor, cognitive, and psychosocial components, and the life-space influences of the activity.

- formulate possible treatment goals that are applicable to the occupational performance areas of work, play, and daily living skills.

- specify modifications which can be made in the activity to increase independent function.

Directions

In preparation for the completion of the Activity Analysis Form (Form 2-5), the student should review the Rationale for the Activity Analysis Process in Chapter 1. The Activity Analysis Form is based on the sequence and the definition of terms as outlined in UTS (see Appendix B). There are four major sections of the Activity Analysis Form, which should be completed according to the guidelines outlined in the following paragraphs:

Part I requires basic information about the activity. This information is to be written in list form beside each item descriptor.

Part II categorizes the components into three sections: sensorimotor, cognitive, and psychosocial. If a skill is necessary to complete the task as it is normally done(see *Purposeful Activity A Position Paper,* Appendix A), the student will indicate the reasoning to the right of the item. If the item is non-applicable or if the skill is not required, the student will write "N/A" to the right of the item and proceed.

Part III addresses the treatment implications of the task and requires treatment goals in each area of occupational performance. Again, the student will indicate his reasoning as described in Part II.

Part IV requires the student to identify appropriate activity modifications which will increase independent function. In this section the student may be asked to assume a dependent role such as performing the activity with the non-dominant hand. As above, the student should indicate his reasoning to the right of each item.

Throughout Parts I, II, and III, it is assumed that the student is performing the activity and the student's own normal responses should be identified, described, and reported. Only the actual performance of the activity described in item A of the Activity Summary should be addressed.

For instance, if the activity described is "pounding a nail into a board," then the student assumes that the hammer, nail and board are gathered together and ready for the activity of pounding a nail. Cutting the board, selecting the nail and going to the tool crib for the hammer were not described as part of the activity. The scope of the activity described in Part I determines the scope of the responses made in Parts II, III, and IV.

Form 2-5 is an example of a blank Activity Analysis form.

Form 2-6 is an example of a completed Activity Analysis form. The Activity Analysis form for completing the assigment is found in Appendix D (Student Worksheets).

Form 2-5.
ACTIVITY ANALYSIS FORM

Student: _____ Date: _____

Course: _____

Part I - Activity Summary
Directions: Respond to the following in list format.

1. Name of activity

2. Brief description of activity

3. Tools/equipment (non-expendable), cost and source

4. Materials/supplies (expendable), cost and source

5. Space/environmental requirements

6. Sequence of major steps; time required to complete each step

7. Precautions (review "Sequence of major steps")

8. Contraindications (review participant's status)

9. Special considerations (age appropriateness, educational requirements, cultural relevance, sexual identification, other)

10. Acceptable criteria for completed project

Form 2-5. (continued)

Part II - Occupational Performance Components
Directions: Indicate the skill components necessary to complete the task (as it is normally done). State your reasoning to the right of each item. Write "N/A" if not applicable. Refer to Uniform Terminology (Appendix B) for definitions of terms.

A. Sensorimotor Components
   1. Neuromuscular
      a. Reflex integration

      b. Range of motion
         (1) active

         (2) passive

         (3) active assistive

      c. Gross and fine coordination
         (1) muscle control

         (2) coordination

         (3) dexterity

      d. Strength and endurance
         (1) building strength, cardiopulmonary reserve

         (2) increasing length of work period

         (3) decreasing fatigue/strain

   2. Sensory integration
      a. Sensory awareness
         (1) tactile awareness

         (2) stereognosis

         (3) kinesthesia

         (4) proprioceptive awareness

         (5) ocular control

         (6) vestibular awareness

         (7) auditory awareness

         (8) gustatory awareness

         (9) olfactory awareness

Form 2-5. (continued)

   b. Visual-spatial awareness
      (1) figure-ground

      (2) form constancy

      (3) position in space

   c. Body integration
      (1) body schema

      (2) postural balance

      (3) bilateral motor coordination

      (4) right-left discrimination

      (5) visual-motor integration

      (6) crossing the midline

      (7) praxis

B. Cognitive Components
   1. Orientation

   2. Conceptualization/comprehension
      a. Concentration

      b. Attention span

      c. Memory

   3. Cognitive integration
      a. Generalization

      b. Problem solving
         (1) defining or evaluating the problem

         (2) organizing a plan

         (3) making decisions/judgment

         (4) implementing a plan

         (5) evaluating decision/judgment

Form 2-5. (continued)

C. Psychosocial Components
   1. Self-management
      a. Self-expression
         (1) experiencing/recognizing a range of emotions

         (2) having an adequate vocabulary

         (3) writing and speaking skills

         (4) use of nonverbal signs and symbols

      b. Self-control
         (1) observing own and others' behavior

         (2) recognizing need for behavior/action change

         (3) imitating new behaviors

         (4) directing energies into stress-reducing behaviors

   2. Dyadic interaction
      a. Understanding norms of communication and interaction

      b. Setting limits on self and others

      c. Compromising and negotiating

      d. Handling stress

      e. Cooperating and competing with others

      f. Responsibly relying on self and others

Form 2-5. (continued)

3. Group interaction
   a. Performing social/emotional roles and tasks

   b. Understanding simple group process

   c. Participating in a mutually beneficial group

D. Task Requirements
   1. Work patterns
      a. Light

      b. Moderate

      c. Heavy

   2. Method
      a. Structured

      b. Methodical

      c. Repetitive

      d. Expressive

      e. Creative

      f. Orderly

      g. Physical contact

      h. Projective

Form 2-5. (continued)

Part III - Occupational Performance
Directions: Indicate possible treatment goals that this activity might address in one or more of the areas of occupational performance. State your reasoning as in Part I. Write "N/A" if not applicable.

A. Independent Living/Daily Living Skills
 1. Physical daily living skills
  a. Grooming and hygiene

  b. Feeding/eating

  c. Dressing

  d. Functional mobility

  e. Functional communication

  f. Object manipulation

 2. Psychological/emotional daily living skills
  a. Self-concept/self-identity

  b. Situational coping

  c. Community involvement

 3. Work
  a. Homemaking

  b. Child care/parenting

  c. Employment preparation

 4. Play/leisure
  a. Recognizing one's needs

  b. Identifying characteristics of play

  c. Selecting play activities

  d. Adaptation of activities

  e. Utilizing community resources

Form 2-5. (continued)

Part IV - Occupational Performance Modifications
Directions: Indicate ways this activity might be modified to increase independent function. State your reasoning. Write "N/A" if not applicable.

Note: This activity should be done with the non-dominant hand only.

A. Therapeutic Adaptations
   1. Orthotics
      a. Static or dynamic positioning

      b. Relief of pain

      c. Maintain joint alignment

      d. Protect joint integrity

      e. Improve function

      f. Decrease deformity

   2. Prosthetics

   3. Assistive/adaptive equipment
      a. Architectural modification

      b. Environmental modification

      c. Assistive equipment

      d. Wheelchair modification

B. Prevention
   1. Energy conservation
      a. Energy-saving procedures

      b. Activity restriction

      c. Work simplification

      d. Time management

      e. Environmental organization

Form 2-5. (continued)

2. Joint protection/body mechanics
   a. Proper body mechanics

   b. Avoiding static/deforming postures

   c. Avoiding excessive weight bearing

   d. Positioning

   e. Coordinating daily living activities

Implications for Treatment

Directions: Explain how and for whom this activity could be beneficial. Indicate physical and/or psychosocial dysfunction.

Grading the Activity

Directions: Describe ways you might grade this activity in terms of:

1. Duration/endurance

2. Range of motion

3. Resistance

4. Complexity

5. Independence

Form 2-6.
ACTIVITY ANALYSIS FORM

Student: _Example_ _____ Date: _____
Course: _____

Part I - Activity Summary
Directions: Respond to the following in list format.

1. Name of activity
   Making a telephone call from a pay phone in a public building.

2. Brief description of activity
   Making a telephone call from a public building requires locating a phone booth, inserting correct change into the coin slot, and pressing the appropriate numbers in order to engage in a conversation with the intended party.

3. Tools/equipment (non-expendable), cost and source
   The equipment required would be a telephone and a telephone book in a public building. There would be no cost to the client for these items.

4. Materials/supplies (expendable), cost and source
   The correct amount of change required would be necessary to place the call. In most locations a local call requires $.25.

5. Space/environmental requirements
   The telephone should be in a private, quiet location.

6. Sequence of major steps; time required to complete each step
   a. *Locate telephone in public building: 2 mins*
   b. *Obtain correct change: 10 secs*
   c. *Lift up the receiver: 2 secs*
   d. *Deposit coin in telephone coin slot: 2 secs*
   e. *Press appropriate numbered buttons when dial tone is heard: 10 secs*
   f. *Wait for answer and engage in conversation: 5 min*

7. Precautions (review "Sequence of major steps")
   In order to avoid a confrontation or assault situation, a defensive posture should be maintained at the phone booth.

8. Contraindications (review participant's status)
   There are no apparent contraindications.

9. Special considerations (age appropriateness, education requirements, cultural relevance, sexual identification, other)
   The ability to problem solve and conceptualize numbers is necessary to complete a telephone call.

10. Acceptable criteria for completed project
    The caller engages in a conversation with the intended party.

Form 2-6. (continued)

Part II - Occupational Performance Components

Directions: Indicate the skill components necessary to complete the task (as it is normally done). State your reasoning to the right of each item. Write "N/A" if not applicable. Refer to Uniform Terminology (Appendix B) for definitions of terms.

A. Sensorimotor Components
 1. Neuromuscular
    a. Reflex integration
       Necessary to allow voluntary, controlled movement to occur
    b. Range of motion
       (1) active
          Necessary to manipulate telephone receiver
       (2) passive
          N/A
       (3) active assistive
          N/A
    c. Gross and fine coordination
       (1) muscle control
          Necessary to coordinate and direct movement in order to place telephone call
       (2) coordination
          Control of muscle groups is necessary to lift and hold receiver and obtain correct change
       (3) dexterity
          Manipulation of wrist and fingers is necessary to push appropriate buttons and deposit coins
    d. Strength and endurance
       (1) building strength, cardiopulmonary reserve
          N/A
       (2) increasing length of work period
          N/A
       (3) decreasing fatigue/strain
          N/A
 2. Sensory integration
    a. Sensory awareness
       (1) tactile awareness
          Needed to distinguish between large and small objects and to identify buttons on phone
       (2) stereognosis
          Needed to manipulate coins, the buttons on phone, and the receiver
       (3) kinesthesia
          Needed to be aware of motion in order to accurately complete call
       (4) proprioceptive awareness
          Needed to perceive position and movement in order to complete call and maintain defensive posture for precautions
       (5) ocular control
          Necessary to locate coins and appropriate buttons and to see what one is doing
       (6) vestibular awareness
          Necessary to maintain posture and balance
       (7) auditory awareness
          Necessary to hear dial tone and engage in conversation

Form 2-6. (continued)

    (8) gustatory awareness
        N/A
    (9) olfactory awareness
        N/A
  b. Visual-spatial awareness
    (1) figure-ground
        Need to discern the required buttons to push from the bank of numbered buttons
    (2) form constancy
        Must recognize phone in a different setting to be consistent with task
    (3) position in space
        Must have knowledge of one's position in space relative to the telephone and public building
  c. Body integration
    (1) body schema
        Necessary to recognize the physical self in reference to the activity
    (2) postural balance
        Required for standing while placing the telephone call
    (3) bilateral motor coordination
        Needed to manipulate receiver and press buttons for smooth and refined completion of task
    (4) right-left discrimination
        N/A
    (5) visual-motor integration
        Must possess eye/hand coordination to allow to push buttons and coin deposits
    (6) crossing midline
        Required while dialing phone number
    (7) praxis
        Motor planning is necessary to achieve purposeful movements required to complete the call

B. Cognitive Components
  1. Orientation
    Must be oriented to time, self, and place in order to place a call
  2. Conceptualization/comprehension
    a. Concentration
      Required for steps necessary to place call and to maintain attention for conversation
    b. Attention span
      Must be able to concentrate long enough to place call and engage in conversation
    c. Memory
      Must remember sequencing of using a telephone
  3. Cognitive integration
    a. Generalization
      Necessary to use phone skills in other locations and with other equipment
    b. Problem solving
      (1) defining or evaluating the problem
        Must be able to determine which numbers to dial and must be able to obtain correct change
      (2) organizing a plan
        Must complete steps in logical, sequenced manner
      (3) making decisions/judgment
        Must make appropriate decisions when obtaining correct change and when engaging in conversation

Form 2-6. (continued)

(4) implementing a plan
Must be able to follow logical steps, such as listen for dial tone before pressing numbers in order to complete call

(5) evaluating decision/judgment
Call completed satisfactorily

C. Psychosocial Components
1. Self-management
   a. Self-expression
      (1) experiencing/recognizing a range of emotions
      Recognition of emotions during conversation of self and intended party
      (2) having an adequate vocabulary
      Necessary to express self and engage in conversation
      (3) writing and speaking skills
      Needs functional speech to be understood by intended party
      (4) use of nonverbal signs and symbols
      Number concept is necessary for completing call, and recognition of telephone sign might be necessary to locate telephone
   b. Self-control
      (1) observing own and others' behaviors
      Necessary to remain in defensive posture because of precautions. Also necessary for conversation with intended party
      (2) recognizing need for behavior/action change
      Must be able to adapt procedure if call cannot be completed
      (3) imitating new behaviors
      N/A
      (4) directing energies into stress-reducing behaviors
      Must be able to control or reduce stress if a stressful situation arises during conversation
2. Dyadic interaction
   a. Understanding norms of communications and interaction
   Must have concept of telephone etiquette to appropriately converse with intended party
   b. Setting limits on self and others
   Must limit conversation time as a courtesy to intended party and others who might be waiting for the telephone
   c. Compromising and negotiating
   Must be able to make conversation compromises if necessary
   d. Handling stress
   Must not become overstressed if conversation is to be productive
   e. Cooperating and competing with others
   Must be cooperative to engage in a dyadic conversation
   f. Responsibly relying on self and others
   Must be confident enough to make a phone call
3. Group interaction
   a. Performing social/emotional roles and tasks
   N/A
   b. Understanding simple group process
   N/A
   c. Participating in a mutually beneficial group
   N/A

Form 2-6. (continued)

D. Task Requirements
1. Work patterns
   a. Light
      Minimal physical work is required
   b. Moderate
      N/A
   c. Heavy
      N/A
2. Method
   a. Structured
      Task requires a structured format
   b. Methodical
      N/A
   c. Repetitive
      N/A
   d. Expressive
      Must be able to express orally to engage in conversation with intended party
   e. Creative
      N/A
   f. Orderly
      N/A
   g. Physical contact
      N/A
   h. Projective
      N/A

Form 2-6. (continued)

Part III - Occupational Performance
Directions: Indicate possible treatment goals that this activity might address in one or more of the areas of occupational performance. State your reasoning as in Part I. Write "N/A" if not applicable.

A. Independent Living/Daily Living Skills
   1. Physical daily living skills
      a. Grooming and hygiene
        N/A
      b. Feeding/eating
        N/A
      c. Dressing
        N/A
      d. Functional mobility
        Manuvering throughout a public building in order to locate a telephone booth enhances functional mobility
      e. Functional communication
        The process of making the call and engaging in the conversation builds and enhances functional communication skills
      f. Object manipulation
        Handling the receiver and the coins would enhance manipulation skills

   2. Psychological/emotional daily living skills
      a. Self-concept/self-identity
        Completion of task aids in enhancing self-concept
      b. Situational coping
        If the line is busy, situational coping will be necessary to proceed
      c. Community involvement

   3. Work
      a. Homemaking
        N/A
      b. Child care/parenting
        N/A
      c. Employment preparation
        N/A

   4. Play/leisure
      a. Recognizing one's needs
        N/A
      b. Identifying characteristics of play
        N/A
      c. Selecting play activities
        N/A
      d. Adaptation of activities
        N/A
      e. Utilizing community resources
        N/A

Form 2-6. (continued)

Part IV - Occupational Performance Modifications
Directions: Indicate ways this activity might be modified to increase independent function. State your reasoning. Write "N/A" if not applicable.

Note: This activity should be done with the non-dominant hand only.

A. Therapeutic Adaptations
  1. Orthotics
     a. Static or dynamic positioning
        N/A
     b. Relief of pain
        N/A
     c. Maintain joint alignment
        N/A
     d. Protect joint integrity
        N/A
     e. Improve function
        N/A
     f. Decrease deformity
        N/A

  2. Prosthetics
     N/A

  3. Assistive/adaptive equipment
     a. Architectural modification
        N/A
     b. Environmental modification
        The telephone booth needs to have a ledge or shelf available for phone book and personal belongings to facilitate access of coins
     c. Assistive equipment
        An adaptive shoulder rest for the telephone receiver would enable the task to be done single handedly.
     d. Wheelchair modification
        N/A

B. Prevention
  1. Energy conservation
     a. Energy-saving procedures
        N/A
     b. Activity restriction
        N/A
     c. Work simplification
        Have telephone number and coins within easy access
     d. Time management
        N/A
     e. Environmental organization
        N/A

Form 2-6. (continued)

2. Joint protection/body mechanics
   a. Proper body mechanics
      N/A
   b. Avoiding static/deforming postures
      Be sure adaptive rest is customized to avoid neck and shoulder pain
   c. Avoiding excessive weight bearing
      N/A
   d. Positioning
      Body positioned for function
   e. Coordination of daily living activities
      N/A

Implications for Treatment

Directions: Explain how and for whom this activity could be beneficial. Indicate physical and/or psychosocial dysfunction.

Physical: This activity would be beneficial to patients with physical dysfunctions by increasing independent function. The manipulation of the objects would increase strength and endurance of the non-dominant hand, making it more functional for other activities. The completion of the task would aid in building self-esteem and encourage more independent functioning as a result. The physical dysfunctions that would benefit would be fractures, short-term upper extremity injuries, amputation, or paralysis.

Psychosocial: Patients with psychosocial dysfunctions would benefit by increasing self-esteem and self-concept. This would also be beneficial for those who have difficulties talking with others. The conversation would provide an opportunity for increasing effective communication. This activity would also aid in increasing attention span and problem-solving skills. The psychosocial dysfunctions that would benefit from this activity would be problems of cognition, memory, speech, sequence and organization, and attention deficit.

Grading the Activity

Directions: Describe ways you might grade this activity in terms of:
1. Duration/endurance
   Time the activity, work toward a decreased time
2. Range of motion
   Adjust the relationship of the individual to the telephone
3. Resistance
   Add weights to arm or telephone receiver
4. Complexity
   Grade call from local to long distance with directory assisted calls
5. Independence
   Decrease assistance as independent functioning increases

Applying the Skills

The Patient-Activity Correlation Form

Rationale

The relationship between the patient's disability and the purposeful activity selected as a therapeutic modality is called the Patient-Activity Correlation (PAC). A positive Patient-Activity Correlation occurs only when the activity produces a response that is significant to the goals of therapy. A negative correlation would occur if the activity produced a harmful response or, at best, no response at all.

The patient's records and the occupational therapy referral coupled with the therapist's expertise lay the foundation for a positive Patient-Activity Correlation. Drawing from the referral and assessment information, the therapist writes a treatment plan that defines the long- and short-term therapy goals.

An important part of the treatment plan is a written expression of the long- and short-term goals by which the therapist will guide the patient through the therapy process. Long-term goals indicate the expected outcome of therapy. They are the objectives of therapy based on the therapist's assessment of the patient's needs. The therapist may project several long-term goals for the patient. Each long-term goal may be comprised of several short-term goals. Short-term goals may be considered as the units of accomplishment that must be completed to reach the long term goals. They are described as the successive building blocks (activity sequenced for improving performance) that become significant components of the treatment plan. As you can see in the following example, one long-term goal is accomplished by four short-term goals.

Long-term goal: The patient will become proficient in his independent dressing skills.

Short-term goal (reflecting the long-term goal): To become proficient in independent dressing, the patient will learn to:

- select appropriate clothing (based on climate, purpose, fit)

- don clothing in sequence (socks first, then shoes)

- arrange clothing appropriately (tuck in the shirt)

- secure fastenings (zip, button, tie)

Both long- and short-term goals must be observable (e.g., the patient can now dress himself independently) and measurable (e.g., within 20 mins), must be supported by theory (e.g., independent living skills), and must be recorded in appropriate documentation using Uniform Terminology (UTS).

Because accountability, efficacy and cost containment are prime criteria for service reimbursement in the current treatment structure, the use of activity must be justifiable. All goals of therapy fall into one or more of the occupational performance areas of daily living skills, work, or play/leisure. UTS defines and describes the outcome of the patient's participation in the activity and documents the use of the activity as a therapeutic modality.

Objectives

The objective of the Patient-Activity Correlation (PAC) form is to direct the student through the treatment sequence portion of the occupational therapy process, moving from the patient profile through the therapeutic application. The occupational therapy process, thoroughly described by Trombly (1983), Reed (1983), Hopkins and Smith (1988) and UTS, basically involves referral, screening, evaluation, planning, implementation, re-evaluation and discharge. The PAC form addresses that portion of the occupational therapy process that moves from referral and evaluation to treatment and documentation (therapeutic application).

The reader should realize that the purpose of the Patient-Activity Correlation is to introduce a framework for treatment, not to teach treatment per se. This framework consists of six sections: patient profile, treatment goals and description of the activity, which includes preparation, implementation and precautions, activity sequence and documentation. The concept of the total treatment plan is wider than the focus of this manual and therefore not addressed at this time.

Upon completion of the Patient-Activity Correlation form, the student will be able to:

- summarize the patient's condition.

- describe long- and short-term goals of therapy.

- select an appropriate activity and prepare for its implementation.

- describe the action steps relevant to therapy.

- document the treatment outcome according to UTS.

Directions

Part 1—Patient Profile The student will summarize the patient's areas of dysfunction and will record those areas that are appropriate for occupational therapy intervention. A patient profile may be assigned by the instructor, read from a chart/referral or found in a text. While the following example addresses physical disability, any dysfunction may be used:

The patient suffered a slash wound to the thenar eminence of the right thumb. The wound has been surgically repaired. The patient is referred to occupational therapy for increase of strength and range of motion, right thumb.

Part 2—Therapeutic Goals From the information gained in Part 1, the student will theorize one long-term goal for the patient and enter it in under Therapeutic Goals (long-term). The student then will write one short-term goal reflecting the long-term goal and enter it under Therapeutic Goals (short-term).

Long-term goal: *The patient will reach maximum strength and range-of-motion through a series of graded activities designed to increase thumb-finger opposition and strength.*
Short-term goal: *The patient will increase muscle strength in the opponens pollicis longus using the pinch method for building with ceramic clay.*

When initially working with the Patient-Activity Correlation Form, the student is asked to formulate only one long-term goal that addresses the patient's needs and then to support that goal with one short-term goal. As the student proceeds academically and clinically, the amount of patient information available to the student will increase and the number of goals (both long- and short-term goals) will increase accordingly.

Part 3—Goal-Directed Activity Description   The student will enter a brief description of the activity, as shown in the following example:

The patient will fashion a small pinch pot from a ball of soft clay by alternately pinching and rotating the clay between his right thumb and fingers. The left hand will assist by holding the clay as it is formed.

Part 4—Activity Preparation Requirements   In addition to formulating the treatment plan, the therapist needs to be prepared to complete the treatment session with a minimum of distraction. Therefore, the therapist is responsible to see that all equipment, materials and treatment modalities are in place before the treatment session begins. For example, conducting a process group may require minimum advanced preparation for the therapist. In contrast, preparation for a treatment session devoted to meal preparation may be more complex in terms of designating and finding equipment, materials, assistive personnel, and a suitable work space. A patient outing can also require a significant period of planning by the therapist. The student will enter this type of information under the Activity Preparation Requirements.

Part 5—Activity Implementation Requirements   During the treatment phase, the therapist will work within a specified time frame. The treatment setting could be in the clinic, at bedside or in the community. The environment may be soothing, neutral or stimulating. The therapist may need the assistance of another staff member or a caregiver, or may cotreat with another professional. The materials and equipment incorporated in the treatment will need to be in place. The therapist will observe safety precautions in relation to the patient's condition as well as that of the therapist and any other assistive personnel. The student will enter this type of information under the Activity Implementation Requirements.

Part 6—Activity Sequence   The student will record the major steps of the activity. It is the major steps that make the activity an appropriate treatment modality, not the incidental ones. If there are more incidental steps than those related specifically to the treatment requirements, the activity should be replaced with a more relevant one. The action steps must be written so that they reflect the stated goals of therapy. This is the essence of purposeful activity.

The student should be aware that only a portion of the activity may be applicable to the treatment. For example, a patient using clay to improve his thumb-finger opposition would not be involved in or responsible for wedging the clay or firing the kiln. Prepared clay of the appropriate amount and resistance would be given to the patient as part of a graded sequence of activity to improve function. Prepared balls of clay will become larger and firmer as the patient's function improves. The progress is documented. With increased clinical experience, the student will be able to refine his observations through the use of specific tests and evaluations. The following example illustrates how an activity sequence could be written:

Example: The patient will:

- hold a 2 to 3 inch diameter ball of soft clay between finger tips and both thumbs firmly

- press both thumbs into top of clay ball simultaneously using thumb-finger opposition

- slightly rotate ball on finger tips as thumbs continue to press clay to within $1/2$ inch of the bottom

- transfer opened ball to left hand

- erase cracks in clay with right thumb and water using a lateral sweeping motion

- continue pressing and smoothing clay with thumb-finger opposition until walls and bottom are of even thickness

- turn pot onto rim to dry

- using thumb-finger opposition, sponge dried pot lightly

It is important to understand that the self-esteem derived from the glazed and fired pot would be of secondary importance here. If the primary goal was to increase self-esteem (as in psychosocial dysfunction) then the thumb-finger strength gained in the activity would be of little consequence.

Part 7—Therapeutic Application: The Uniform Terminology System (UTS) The final section of the patient-activity correlation is the documentation of the activity as a therapeutic modality. The student will complete this section by designating under which areas of UTS the steps of the activity fall. The student will review the patient profile, the therapy goals, the activity description and the action steps. Using UTS, the results of the treatment intervention are documented by recording the occupational performance area (daily living skill, work, or play/leisure) and the performance components addressed. The documentation should directly reflect the requirements of the referral. If the referral required increased range of motion, the UTS should indicate that increased range of motion was addressed. Moving through a full circle, the referral information will generate goals; goals will demand activity; activity response will be documented by UTS; and, finally, the documentation should confirm that the referral has been addressed through occupational therapy intervention. The following examples present these Uniform Terminology areas addressed by the clay pinch pot activity. Notice that the number and letter designations correspond to the actual organization of the first edition of the UTS (Appendix B).

The student should understand that one therapeutic application may address several steps of the activity sequence. Sometimes a whole series of steps will be addressed by one performance area or component. Through the language of UTS, the use of the activity to attain a treatment outcome is documented and thereby achieves credibility as a treatment modality.

OT Treatment
A. Independent Living/Daily Living Skills (Occupational Performance Area)
    3. Work
        c. Employment preparation
           (3) work skills and performance
A. Sensorimotor Components (Occupational Performance Components)
    1. Neuromuscular
        b. Range of motion
           (1) active
        c. Gross and fine coordination
           (1) muscle control
           (3) dexterity
        d. Strength and endurance

By way of review, the process of utilizing an activity as a therapeutic modality has been presented in four phases. In the first phase, the student became aware that there can be more to an activity than simply doing it (Activity Awareness). In the second phase, the student sequentially dissected the activity to reveal its individual segments (Action Identification). In the Activity Analysis phase, the student examined the sensorimotor, cognitive, and psychosocial occupational performance components and was encouraged to consider and record all the possible applications that an activity may contribute as a therapeutic modality. In the Patient-Activity Correlation phase, the student addressed a long- and short-term treatment goal of a specific patient from using the activity described. The outcome of the recorded action steps was then documented through the use of UTS (See Figure 2-3).

Form 2-7 is an example of a blank Patient-Activity Correlation form.

Form 2-8 is an example of a completed Patient-Activity Correlation form. The Patient Activity form for completing the assignment is found in Appendix D (Student Worksheets).

Form 2-7.
PATIENT-ACTIVITY CORRELATION FORM

Student: _____

Course: _____ Date: _____

1. Patient Profile

2. Therapeutic Goals
   a. Long Term

   b. Short Term

3. Goal-Directed Activity Description

4. Activity Preparation Requirements
   a. Task

   b. Personnel

   c. Preparation time

   d. Place/space

   e. Materials

   f. Equipment

   g. Safety precautions (personnel)

Form 2-7. (continued)

5. Activity Implementation Requirements
   a. Personnel

   b. Setting/location

   c. Area/space

   d. Environment

   e. Materials

   f. Equipment/adaptations

   g. Time frame

   h. Safety precautions (patient)

6. Activity Sequence (Action steps: ten or less)

7. Therapeutic Applications (UTS)

Form 2-8.
PATIENT-ACTIVITY CORRELATION FORM

Student: _____

Course: _____ Date: _____

1. Patient Profile
   The client suffered a neck fracture 1 year ago. He is a 20-year-old student who uses a wheelchair. He can transfer independently. He was referred to occupational therapy for increased functional mobility throughout his community. The client needs to be able to telephone for transportation home from school.

2. Therapeutic Goals
   a. Long-Term
      The patient will reach maximum independence through a series of graded activities designed to enable patient to get home from school independently.

   b. Short-Term
      In view of the long-term goal, the patient will independently call for a cab to pick him up at school and drive him home.

3. Goal-Directed Activity Description
   The client will use a pay telephone in a public building to access transportation (a cab).

4. Activity Preparation Requirements
   a. Task
      N/A

   b. Personnel
      One therapist

   c. Preparation time
      Approximately 1 hour

   d. Place/space
      Public building that is wheelchair accessible with an accessible public telephone

   e. Materials
      N/A

   f. Equipment
      N/A

   g. Safety precautions (personnel)
      N/A

Form 2-8. (continued)

5. Activity Implementation Requirements
   a. Personnel
   N/A

   b. Setting/location
   N/A

   c. Area/space
   Public building with telephone that is wheelchair accessible

   d. Environment
   Quiet surroundings with privacy for the learning process

   e. Materials
   N/A

   f. Equipment/adaptations
   None

   g. Time frame
   N/A

   h. Safety precautions (patient)
   Maintain posture and balance for stability for prevent further injury

6. Activity Sequence (Action steps: ten or less)
   a. Locate public telephone and note location
   b. Stabilize wheelchair
   c. Retrieve change for telephone
   d. Pick up receiver
   e. Deposit coins in telephone lots
   f. Press appropriate numbers
   g. Make arrangements for pick-up, relaying location and estimated time of arrival
   h. Hang up receiver
   i. Transport to pick-up point

7. Therapeutic Application (UTS)

   INDEPENDENT LIVING/DAILY LIVING SKILLS
   Physical daily living skills
   Functional mobility
   Functional communication
   Object manipulation

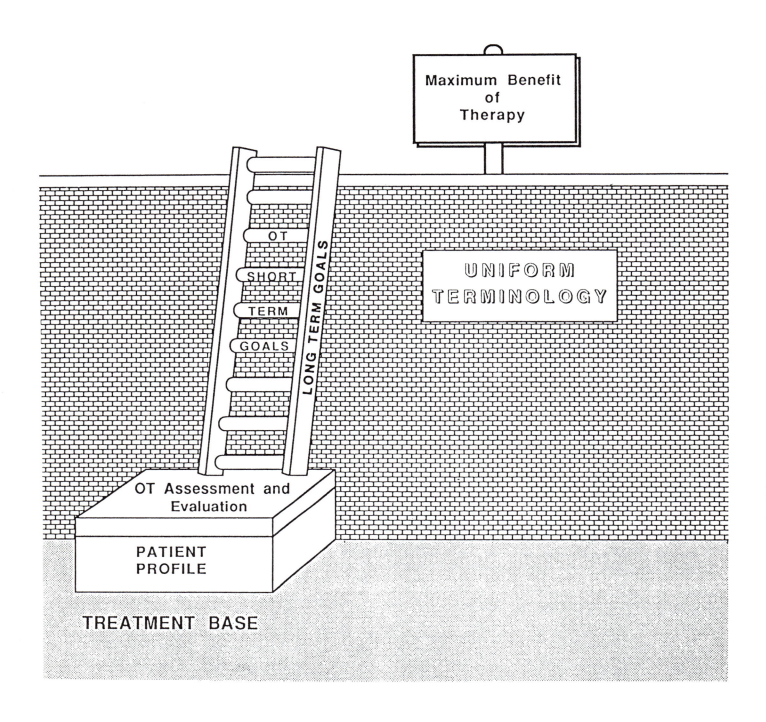

Figure 2-3.

The therapist works from a treatment base of theory, practice, and experience.
Upon receiving a patient profile (the referral for occupational therapy services and the patient history),
the therapist proceeds with appropriate assessments and/or evaluations. Following the evaluative
process the therapist writes a treatment plan that includes the long- and short-term goals that will
progress the patient towards maximum benefit of therapy. This process is described through the use of
uniform terminology.

References

Center for Learning Resources. (1979). *T.A.S.K. A.C.T.: A Pre-instructional analysis process. Teaching improvement systems for health care educators.* Lexington, KY: University of Kentucky.

Crepeau, E.L. (1986). *Activity Programming for the Elderly.* Boston: Little, Brown & Co.

Hopkins, H.L. & Smith, H.D. (1988). *Willard and Spackman's Occupational Therapy, Seventh Edition.* Philadelphia: J.B. Lippincott Co.

Reed, K. & Sanderson, S. (1983). *Concepts of Occupational Therapy, Second Edition.* Baltimore: Williams & Wilkins.

Reilly, M. (1962). Occupational therapy can be one of the great ideas of 20th century medicine. *The American Journal of Occupational Therapy, 16*(1), 1-9.

Rogers, J.C. (1982). The spirit of independence: The education of a philosophy. *The American Journal of Occupational Therapy, 36*(11), 709-715.

Ryan, S. (1986). *The Certified Occupational Therapy Assistant.* Thorofare: SLACK Incorporated.

Trombly, C. (1983). *Occupational Therapy for Physical Dysfunction.* Baltimore: Williams & Wilkins.

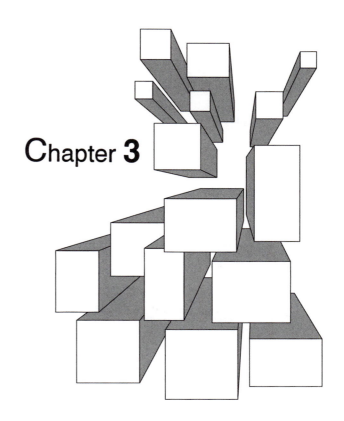

Chapter 3

ILLUSTRATING THE PROCESS

Application and Examination

Introduction

Rationale
This chapter is designed to further illustrate the process of integrating the therapeutic essence of activity into the regimen of occupational therapy treatment. It consists of completed student samples of Activity Analysis and Patient-Activity Correlation forms which are paired through the application and examination of a single activity.

Activity Analysis
Working in small groups, the students took the assigned task through the process of activity analysis. Each task was simple and familiar so that the students could focus on the task components, not variations on implementation.

The students completed Parts I, II, and III of the Activity Analysis as they themselves normally performed the task. In Part IV, the Occupational Performance Modification, the students responded as though they performed the activity using only the non-dominant hand.

Patient-Activity Correlation

With the activity analysis completed, each student group received a patient profile and a referral for occupational therapy intervention. The students mentally assessed their patient and then formulated one long-term goal and one short-term goal for therapy. The short-term goal reflects the long-term goal and incorporates the task examined in the activity analysis as a treatment modality. In this way, the student crossed the bridge from simple task to purposeful activity and occupational performance.

The experienced reader of Patient-Activity Correlations will immediately see further long- and short-term goals that the activity could address. For the beginning student who is working on developing the concept of long- and short-term goals, one of each is sufficient, although some beginning students may feel comfortable enough with the concept to include several short-term goals.

Objectives
Upon review of this section the student will be able to:

- integrate the process by which an activity can become a treatment modality, and

- apply the concept of purposeful activity to any area of occupational therapy practice.

Sample Paired Activity Analyses and Patient-Activity Correlations
The following samples of assignments and profiles can be used for class discussion or as a suggestion for further assignments. The instructor/student is encouraged to modify or elaborate on any part of these examples. They are the basis for the student samples that follow.

Activity Analysis Assignments
1. Playing beachball with two friends (paired with PAC Profile 1)
2. Washing socks in the bathroom sink (paired with PAC Profile 2)
3. Painting a bedroom wall (paired with PAC Profile 3)
4. Washing dishes in the sink (paired with PAC Profile 4)
5. Making a turkey sandwich (paired with PAC Profile 5)
6. Sewing a button on a shirt (paired with PAC Profile 6)

Patient-Activity Correlation Profiles
1. Johnny Adkins is a 10-year-old male with learning disabilities. An evaluation by the school occupational therapist indicates deficits in depth perception, ocular control and proprioception, and bilateral incoordination. Johnny is shy around his class-mates and he is easily frustrated. Johnny has been referred to occupational therapy for treatment following the recommendations discussed during his school case conferences.
2. Mary and Joe Wells are young adults who have joined a travel group sponsored by United Cerebral Palsy of Indiana. Both have spastic cerebral palsy and use wheel-chairs. They have been married approximately one year. This is their first major trip. The group will travel by plane to Disney World in Orlando. Each traveler may take one suitcase. The group has been referred to the occupational therapist to assist them with the selection and care of lightweight, easy-care clothing for travel.
3. Wendy Jenkins is a 15-year-old female with a diagnosis of oppositional defiance disorder. Wendy is openly defiant with her parents and teachers. She states that they won't let her express her feelings and that they "boss her too much." Patient has

been referred to occupational therapy for assessment and treatment in terms of activities that will permit Wendy to have control within specific areas of space and time without adult intervention.

4. Alice Murphy is a 47-year-old female with a diagnosis of rheumatoid arthritis, primarily affecting the upper extremities. She also experiences pain and stiffness in her knees in the morning. She finds that managing her house is becoming more difficult as her disease progresses. Patient has been referred to occupational therapy for assessment and treatment for homemaking skills, joint protection, and energy conservation.

5. George Handley is a 76-year-old male who has been attending a senior citizen's center since his wife died two months ago. His wife did all the cooking and homemaking in which the client participated very little. Mr. Handley comes to the center for socialization and a full, hot meal at noon. He returns to his small home about 4:30 PM. He travels by bus. During the noon meal he stated that he seldom has supper because it is too much trouble and because he hasn't had too much experience in the kitchen. He is noticeably thinner than when he first came to the center. Patient has been referred to the home health therapist for evaluation and treatment for kitchen skills and safety as well as increased motivation for eating.

6. Mike Marshall is a 19-year-old male with a diagnosis of moderate mental retardation. The client has been referred to occupational therapy for work preparation and self-care skills. He has progressed and is now ready to move from his parents' home to a group home where he will be responsible for all his self-care which includes arriving at his job site in clean, neat and appropriate clothing. Patient has been referred to occupational therapy for assessment and treatment of self-care and job-readiness skills.

Acknowledgment:

The Indiana University Occupational Therapy Baccalaureate Class of 1993 contributed wholly or in part to the Activity Analysis and Patient-Activity Correlations used in Chapter 3. Examples used by permission.

Form 3-1.
ACTIVITY ANALYSIS FORM

Student: *Example* _____ Date: _____

Course: _____

Part I - Activity Summary
Directions: Respond to the following in list format.

1. Name of activity
   Playing beach ball with two friends

2. Brief description of activity
   Friend #1 will toss the ball to friend #2. Friend #2 will toss the ball to friend #3. Friend #3 will toss the ball back to friend #1. Keep repeating the process.

3. Tools/equipment (nonexpendable), cost and source
   Beach ball—$2.50, K-mart

4. Materials/supplies (expendable), cost and source
   None

5. Space/environmental requirements
   An open space is needed to toss the ball freely without hitting surrounding objects or people. For full enjoyment, when playing with a beach ball, a beach is needed.

6. Sequence of major steps: time required for each step
   a. *Friend #1 holds the ball with flexed arms: 2 sec.*
   b. *Friend #1 steps out and extends arms forcefully: 2 sec.*
   c. *Friend #1 releases ball simultaneously: 5 sec.*
   d. *Friend #2 located ball visually: 2 sec.*
   e. *Friend #2 makes contact with ball with partially extended arms: 5 sec.*
   f. *Friend #2 secures ball with hands and flexes arms: 1 sec.*
   g. *Friend #2 excitedly prepares to repeat process with friend #1: 2 sec.*

7. Precautions (review "Sequence of major steps")
   Make sure that there are no people in area that could be hit by beach ball. Avoid strong winds, and be careful not to get sand in eyes.

8. Contraindications (review participant's status)
   This activity should not be undertaken in bad weather. Also, an injury which would cause pain when tossing the ball would make the activity inappropriate. Sun sensitivity should be considered.

9. Special considerations (age appropriateness, educational requirements, cultural relevance, sexual identification, other)
   Weather should be appropriate; extreme temperatures and dangerous weather should be avoided.

10. Acceptable criteria for completed project
    Everyone has had fun, is tired, and has had his or her turn.

Form 3-1. (continued)

Part II - Occupational Performance Components
Directions: Indicate the skill components necessary to complete the task (as it is normally done). State your reasoning to the right of each item. Write "N/A" if not applicable. Refer to Uniform Terminology (Appendix B) for definitions of terms.

A. Sensorimotor Components
1. Neuromuscular
   a. Reflex integration
      Necessary for voluntary controlled movement
   b. Range of motion
      (1) active
         Necessary to toss the ball independently
      (2) passive
         N/A
      (3) active assistive
         N/A
   c. Gross and fine coordination
      (1) muscle control
         Necessary to direct and grade the force of throw
      (2) coordination
         Enables one to catch and throw ball
      (3) dexterity
         Necessary to grasp the ball
   d. Strength and endurance
      (1) building strength, cardiopulmonary reserve
         Minimal amount of strength needed; occurs only with vigorous play
      (2) increasing length of work period
         N/A
      (3) decreasing fatigue/strain
         Fatigue decreases with each consecutive experience of regular exercise
2. Sensory integration
   a. Sensory awareness
      (1) tactile awareness
         Needed to feel the ball in order to catch it and hold it
      (2) stereognosis
         N/A
      (3) kinesthesia
         Knowing how body is moving is necessary to throw and catch ball
      (4) proprioceptive awareness
         Necessary to know where self is in relation to ball and friends playing
      (5) ocular control
         Necessary to locate the ball visually to throw it and catch it
      (6) vestibular awareness
         Necessary to maintain posture and balance
      (7) auditory awareness
         N/A
      (8) gustatory awareness
         N/A
      (9) olfactory awareness
         N/A

Form 3-1. (continued)

b. Visual-spatial awareness
   (1) figure-ground
       Needed to find ball in space to catch it
   (2) form constancy
       Necessary to recognize the ball
   (3) position in space
       Must know where body is in relation to other objects
c. Body integration
   (1) body schema
       Necessary to be aware of body
   (2) postural balance
       Necessary to ensure balance
   (3) bilateral motor coordination
       Both hands needed for grasping and tossing ball
   (4) right-left discrimination
       N/A
   (5) visual-motor integration
       Hand-eye coordination is required
   (6) crossing the midline
       Needed to throw ball in different directions
   (7) praxis
       Needed to successfully perform activity—to know process of tossing and what you do next

B. Cognitive Components
   1. Orientation
      Must be oriented to place and what is being done there
   2. Conceptualization/comprehension
      a. Concentration
         Necessary to make contact with ball
      b. Attention span
         Necessary to be thinking about game and know when to catch and throw the ball
      c. Memory
         Must remember the process and the order turns are being taken
   3. Cognitive integration
      a. Generalization
         Can be generalized to other types of ball playing
      b. Problem solving
         (1) defining or evaluating the problem
             Deciding who is going to throw to whom
         (2) organizing a plan
             Continue in a sequential manner
         (3) making decisions/judgment
             Decide who's throwing to whom
         (4) implementing a plan
             Following the steps to toss ball
         (5) evaluating decision/judgment
             Determine if task was successful

Form 3-1. (continued)

C. Psychosocial Components
1. Self-management
a. Self-expression
(1) experiencing/recognizing a range of emotions
Should be happy and having fun
(2) having an adequate vocabulary
N/A
(3) writing and speaking skills
N/A
(4) use of nonverbal signs and symbols
When partner prepares to throw, prepare to catch
b. Self-control
(1) observing own and others' behaviors
One must observe appropriate way to throw and to catch
(2) recognizing need for behavior/action change
Modifies if throws ball too hard to too soft
(3) imitating new behaviors
N/A
(4) directing energies into stress-reducing behaviors
N/A

2. Dyadic interaction
a. Understanding norms of communication and interaction
N/A
b. Setting limits on self and others
N/A
c. Compromising and negotiating
N/A
d. Handling stress
N/A
e. Cooperating and competing with others
N/A
f. Responsibly relying on self and others
N/A

3. Group interaction
a. Performing social/emotional roles and tasks
Necessary to share the ball, keep conversation flowing, and be considerate
b. Understanding simple group process
Necessary to know how to take turns, share, and cooperate
c. Participating in a mutually beneficial group
Make sure everyone takes turns and has a good time

Form 3-1. (continued)

D. Task Requirements
  1. Work patterns
     a. Light
        Minimal physical work/strength is required

     b. Moderate
        N/A

     c. Heavy
        N/A

  2. Method
     a. Structured
        One person throws to the next and this pattern should be followed

     b. Methodical
        N/A

     c. Repetitive
        The game continues with repetition of each player taking their turn

     d. Expressive
        N/A

     e. Creative
        N/A

     f. Orderly
        N/A

     g. Physical contact
        Player makes contact with the ball

     h. Projective
        N/A

Form 3-1. (continued)

Part III - Occupational Performance
Directions: Indicate possible treatment goals that this activity might address in one or more of the areas of occupational performance. State your reasoning as in Part I. Write "N/A" if not applicable.

A. Independent Living/Daily Living Skills
    1. Physical daily living skills
        a. Grooming and hygiene
          N/A
        b. Feeding/eating
          N/A
        c. Dressing
          N/A
        d. Functional mobility
          N/A
        e. Functional communication
          N/A
        f. Object manipulation
          N/A

    2. Psychological/emotional daily living skills
        a. Self-concept/self-identity
          N/A
        b. Situational coping
          N/A
        c. Community involvement
          N/A

    3. Work
        a. Homemaking
          N/A
        b. Child care/parenting
          N/A
        c. Employment preparation
          N/A

    4. Play/leisure
        a. Recognizing one's needs
          Necessary for releasing stress, hostility, or excess energy
        b. Identifying characteristics of play
          Nonstressful, friends doing it for fun and relaxation
        c. Selecting play activities
          N/A
        d. Adaptation of activities
          The ball should be vollied to each player rather than tossed, or catch ball in a basket
        e. Utilizing community resources
          N/A

Form 3-1. (continued)

Part IV - Occupational Performance Modifications
Directions: Indicate ways this activity might be modified to increase independent function. State your reasoning. Write "N/A" if not applicable.

Note: This activity should be done with the non-dominant hand only.

A. Therapeutic Adaptations
   1. Orthotics
      a. Static or dynamic positioning
         N/A
      b. Relieve pain
         N/A
      c. Maintain joint alignment
         N/A
      d. Protect joint integrity
         N/A
      e. Improve function
         N/A
      f. Decrease deformity
         N/A

   2. Prosthetics
      N/A

   3. Assistive/adaptive equipment
      a. Architectural modification
         N/A
      b. Environmental modification
         N/A
      c. Assistive equipment
         Use a basket or mitt to catch ball
      d. Wheelchair modification
         N/A

B. Prevention
   1. Energy conservation
      a. Energy-saving procedures
         Taking breaks so as not to strain arm
      b. Activity restriction
         N/A
      c. Work simplification
         Have players stand closer together
      d. Time management
         N/A
      e. Environmental organization
         N/A

Form 3-1. (continued)

2. Joint protection/body mechanics
   a. Proper body mechanics
      Player must be aware of body movements
   b. Avoiding static/deforming postures
      N/A
   c. Avoiding excessive weight bearing
      N/A
   d. Positioning
      Player should work on optimal positioning
   e. Coordinating daily activities
      N/A

Implications for Treatment
Directions: Explain how and for whom this activity could be beneficial. Indicate physical and/or psychosocial dysfunction.

Physical: Strengthens extremities with mild physical exercise. Activity is good for the cardiovascular system and also helps improve hand-eye coordination and equilibrium.

Psychosocial: Activity improves group processes and also works well as a stress reliever. The task also implements learning sequences or patterns by volleying.

Grading the Activity
Directions: Describe ways you might grade this activity in terms of:

1. Duration/endurance
   Begin with short intervals of play, working toward longer intervals of play

2. Range of motion
   Vary the distance between the players

3. Resistance
   Use a weight on the arm

4. Complexity
   Set differing distances and sequences of play

5. Independence
   Give each person a choice of whom to throw ball to

Form 3-1a.
PATIENT-ACTIVITY CORRELATION FORM

Student: _Example (based on Profile 1 – Johnny Adkins)_

Course: _____ Date: _____

1. **Patient Profile**
   Johnny is a 10-year-old male patient who has learning disabilities. His deficits lie in the areas of depth perception, ocular control, proprioception, and bilateral incoordination. Johnny is shy and easily frustrated, and has been referred to occupational therapy for help in dealing with these problems.

2. **Therapeutic Goals**
   a. **Long-term**
      To gain the skill of bilateral coordination

   b. **Short-term**
      To increase bilateral coordination, the client will learn to play catch with a ball with two friends

3. **Goal-Directed Activity Description**
   The patient and friends will start by sitting or crouching on the floor and bouncing the ball back and forth to each other. The more skill gained, the more difficult the activity can be graded so they end up standing playing catch.

4. **Activity Preparation Requirements**
   a. **Task**
      _N/A_

   b. **Personnel**
      The therapist can work alone

   c. **Preparation time**
      The therapist may need approximately 15 min. to inflate the ball and clear an open area to play on

   d. **Place/space**
      The therapist needs to clear a large, flat, open area approximately 9 ft. ✕ 9 ft.

   e. **Materials**
      _N/A_

   f. **Equipment**
      _N/A_

   g. **Safety precautions (personnel)**
      _N/A_

Form 3-1a. (continued)

5. Activity Implementation Requirements
   a. Personnel
      N/A

   b. Setting/location
      N/A

   c. Area/space
      This activity can be carried out on the floor in a large, flat, open area

   d. Environment
      A quiet room is needed where there will be no distractions to allow for optimal concentration

   e. Materials
      N/A

   f. Equipment/adaptations
      Inflatable ball

   g. Time frame
      N/A

   h. Safety/precautions (patient)
      The therapist needs to ensure the patient avoids frustration by having him start with extremely easy tasks first. It is important not to work for too long and to allow for a break if necessary. It is important to make therapy fun, and to provide encouragement.

6. Activity Sequence (Action steps: ten or less)
   a. *Player #1 will visually locate player #2*
   b. *Player #1 will slowly and fully extend arms and thrust the ball to player #2*
   c. *Player #2 will locate the ball visually*
   d. *Player #2 will extend arms to reach for the ball*
   e. *Player #2 will grasp the ball with both hands*
   f. *Player #2 will flex arms to pull the ball in while holding it*
   g. *Player #2 will then repeat the process with player #3, player #3 to player #1, and so on*

7. Therapeutic Application
   INDEPENDENT LIVING/DAILY LIVING SKILLS
     Physical daily living skills
       Functional mobility
       Object manipulation

   SENSORIMOTOR COMPONENTS
     Neuromuscular
       Gross and fine coordination
         muscle control
         coordination
         dexterity
       Strength/endurance
     Sensory integration
       Body integration
         bilateral motor coordination

Form 3-2.
ACTIVITY ANALYSIS FORM

Student: _Example_ _____ Date: _____

Course: _____

Part I - Activity Summary
Directions: Respond to the following in list format.

1. Name of activity
   Washing out socks in the bathroom sink.

2. Brief description of activity
   The student will need to pour soap into the sink, add water forcefully to produce suds, wash the socks until clean, drain the dirty water, and rinse the socks in clean water.

3. Tools/equipment (nonexpendable), cost and source
   The equipment that is needed is a sink and a faucet which should both be located in the bathroom.

4. Materials/supplies (expendable), cost and source
   The materials needed are soap and water. The cost for a small bottle of Woolite is around $3.

5. Space/environmental requirements
   A 3 ft. × 3 ft. space in the bathroom is needed. In this space there must be adequate room for standing, a sink, and a small countertop on which to set the soap.

6. Sequence of major steps: time required for each step
   a. *Plug the sink completely: 2 sec.*
   b. *Pour soap into sink sparingly: 10 sec.*
   c. *Add water forcefully into the sink: 45 sec.*
   d. *Toss socks into water leisurely: 3 sec.*
   e. *Knead socks vigorously: 1 min.*
   f. *Wring out socks completely: 20 sec.*
   g. *Empty sink thoroughly: 30 sec.*
   h. *Rinse socks underwater quickly: 2 min.*
   i. *Wring out socks completely: 20 sec.*
   j. *Lay out socks horizontally to dry: 10 sec.*

7. Precautions (review "Sequence of major steps")
   The student should be careful not to touch the eyes or mouth because this may cause ingestion of soap or burning to the eyes. It is necessary to test the water to assure that the temperature is comfortable to the student's touch.

8. Contraindications (review participant's status)
   This activity would not be beneficial if the student had a burn or open wound on his/her hand. This activity would not be appropriate if the student had an allergy to soap.

9. Special considerations (age appropriateness, educational requirements, cultural relevance, sexual identification, other)
   This activity is appropriate for the student as far as age appropriateness, educational requirements, cultural relevance, and sexual identification.

10. Acceptable criteria for completed project
    If the stains, smell, and soap have been washed out of the socks, then the activity has been completed and the socks are clean.

Form 3-2. (continued)

Part II - Occupational Performance Components

Directions: Indicate the skill components necessary to complete the task (as it is normally done). State your reasoning to the right of each item. Write "N/A" if not applicable. Refer to Uniform Terminology (Appendix B) for definitions of terms.

A. Sensorimotor Components
  1. Neuromuscular
    a. Reflex integration
      If the temperature of the water is uncomfortable to the hands, then reflexes are necessary to withdraw the hands quickly
    b. Range of motion
      (1) active
        Range of motion in the wrists and fingers is used to wash and wring the socks
      (2) passive
        N/A
      (3) active assistive
        N/A
    c. Gross and fine coordination
      (1) muscle control
        Necessary to be able to move the entire body in an appropriate manner for washing out the socks
      (2) coordination
        Must have control over the large muscle groups of arms and shoulders to move the socks up and down in the water
      (3) dexterity
        Need to have control over the small muscles in the fingers to be able to wring the socks out
    d. Strength and endurance
      (1) building strength, cardiopulmonary reserve
        N/A
      (2) increasing length of work period
        N/A
      (3) decreasing fatigue/strain
        N/A
  2. Sensory integration
    a. Sensory awareness
      (1) tactile awareness
        Necessary when trying to locate socks in the soapy water and needed to be able to distinguish if there is soap still left in the socks
      (2) stereognosis
        Discerns an object in the water when the objects are not visible
      (3) kinesthesia
        Helps to determine the amount of force being put on the socks and the motion of rubbing the socks together
      (4) proprioceptive awareness
        Necessary to know how far away the sink or soap is, and to know the position for standing as the socks are being washed
      (5) ocular control
        Used to visually track the socks as they are taken out of the water

Form 3-2. (continued)

(6) vestibular awareness
Balance is necessary in order to stand while wringing out the socks

(7) auditory awareness
N/A

(8) gustatory awareness
N/A

(9) olfactory awareness
N/A

b. Visual-spatial awareness

(1) figure-ground
Needed to be able to distinguish the socks and the soap from the sink

(2) form constancy
Needed to be able to recognize the socks, whether on the sink, in the sink, or on the drying rack

(3) position in space
Allows judgement of how far away the sink is and where the soap is in relation to the student

c. Body integration

(1) body schema
Realizing the hands are being rubbed together and where the hands are in relation to each other

(2) postural balance
Necessary when standing during this activity

(3) bilateral motor coordination
Necessary for manipulating both hands at the same time

(4) right-left discrimination
N/A

(5) visual-motor integration
Hand-eye coordination is needed to rub and wring the socks

(6) crossing the midline
Reaching across the midline to turn on the faucet or to reach the soap

(7) praxis
Necessary for planning the movements in order to complete the task

B. Cognitive Components

1. Orientation
Need to orient self and realize location in the bathroom

2. Conceptualization/comprehension

a. Concentration
A limited amount of concentration is needed to complete the task

b. Attention span
Since the entire process takes only a short time, a limited attention span is needed also

c. Memory
It is necessary to remember which steps are needed to wash the socks, the order in which they appear, and which steps have already been completed

3. Cognitive Integration

a. Generalization
Necessary to be able to generalize from washing socks to washing a shirt. Also needed to generalize from washing one pair of socks to washing two pairs of socks

Form 3-2. (continued)

  b. Problem solving
   (1) defining or evaluating the problem
   Need to decide that the socks are dirty
   (2) organizing a plan
   Need a plan to determine the order of events
   (3) making decisions/judgment
   Need to decide how much soap, water, and time is needed. Also must decide if the temperature is comfortable to the touch
   (4) implementing a plan
   Must be able to carry out the plan
   (5) evaluating decision/judgment
   Must be able to judge when the socks are clean and when they are free of soap

C. Psychosocial Components
  1. Self-management
   a. Self-expression
    (1) experiencing/recognizing a range of emotions
    N/A
    (2) having an adequate vocabulary
    N/A
    (3) writing and speaking skills
    N/A
    (4) use of nonverbal signs and symbols
    N/A
   b. Self-control
    (1) observing own and others' behaviors
    N/A
    (2) recognizing need for behavior/action change
    Recognizes the need to change the way the socks are being washed if they do not come clean
    (3) imitating new behaviors
    N/A
    (4) directing energies into stress-reducing behaviors
    May use the wringing to reduce stress
  2. Dyadic interaction
   a. Understanding norms of communication and interaction
   N/A
   b. Setting limits on self and others
   N/A
   c. Compromising and negotiating
   N/A
   d. Handling stress
   N/A
   e. Cooperating and competing with others
   N/A
   f. Responsibly relying on self and others
   N/A

Form 3-2. (continued)

3. Group interaction
   a. Performing social/emotional roles and tasks
      N/A
   b. Understanding simple group process
      N/A
   c. Participating in a mutually beneficial group
      N/A

D. Task Requirements
   1. Work patterns
      a. Light
         The socks do not weigh much at all and the task does not require great amounts of physical strength
      b. Moderate
         N/A
      c. Heavy
         N/A
   2. Method
      a. Structured
         A particular sequence of events is followed
      b. Methodical
         A procedure is needed in order to wash the socks
      c. Repetitive
         The wringing and the rubbing are both repetitive
      d. Expressive
         N/A
      e. Creative
         N/A
      f. Orderly
         Need to be neat so that water and soap are not accidentally splashed onto the floor
      g. Physical contact
         N/A
      h. Projective
         N/A

Form 3-2. (continued)

Part III - Occupational Performance
Directions: Indicate possible treatment goals that this activity might address in one or more of the areas of occupational performance. State your reasoning as in Part I. Write "N/A" if not applicable.

A. Independent Living/Daily Living Skills
   1. Physical daily living skills
       a. Grooming and hygiene
           Necessary to have clean socks in order to have proper hygiene
       b. Feeding/eating
           N/A
       c. Dressing
           Necessary in order to have proper dress either because it is cold or because the socks are fashionable with the outfit
       d. Functional mobility
           N/A
       e. Functional communication
           N/A
       f. Object manipulation
           Need to manipulate the socks to get them clean

   2. Psychological/emotional daily living skills
       a. Self-concept/self-identity
           N/A
       b. Situational coping
           N/A
       c. Community involvement
           N/A

   3. Work
       a. Homemaking
           N/A
       b. Child care/parenting
           N/A
       c. Employment preparation
           N/A

   4. Play/leisure
       a. Recognizing one's needs
           N/A
       b. Identifying characteristics of play
           N/A
       c. Selecting play activities
           N/A
       d. Adaptation of activities
           N/A
       e. Utilizing community resources
           N/A

Form 3-2. (continued)

Part IV - Occupational Performance Modifications
Directions: Indicate ways this activity might be modified to increase independent function. State your reasoning. Write "N/A" if not applicable.

Note: This activity should be done with the non-dominant hand only.

A. Therapeutic Adaptations
1. Orthotics
   a. Static or dynamic positioning
      N/A
   b. Relieve pain
      N/A
   c. Maintain joint alignment
      N/A
   d. Protect joint integrity
      N/A
   e. Improve function
      N/A
   f. Decrease deformity
      N/A

2. Prosthetics
   N/A

3. Assistive/adaptive equipment
   a. Architectural modification
      N/A
   b. Environmental modification
      N/A
   c. Assistive equipment
      Small washboard for rubbing socks on may be useful, but not mandatory
   d. Wheelchair modification
      N/A

B. Prevention
1. Energy conservation
   a. Energy-saving procedures
      Taking all materials to the sink in one trip or leaving them in the bathroom
   b. Activity restriction
      N/A
   c. Work simplification
      N/A
   d. Time management
      Washing all pairs of dirty socks in the same time period
   e. Environmental organization
      Keeping the washboard and soap in the bathroom

Form 3-2. (continued)

2. Joint protection/body mechanics
   a. Proper body mechanics
      N/A
   b. Avoiding static/deforming postures
      Use good posture whether sitting or standing during the activity
   c. Avoiding excessive weight bearing
      N/A
   d. Positioning
      Position chair close to sink
   e. Coordinating daily living skills
      N/A

Implications for Treatment
Directions: Explain how and for whom this activity could be beneficial. Indicate physical and/or psychosocial dysfunction.

Physical: Washing socks out in the sink could be used with patients who have problems with range of motion, hand or finger dexterity, and decreased motor control in the upper extremities, especially those with fine motor control problems, in addition to stroke and cerebral palsy patients and patients with a neuromuscular disorder.

Psychosocial: Washing socks out in the bathroom sink could be used for patients who have a short attention span to increase this; patients with problems in the ability to plan or problem solve; and the mentally retarded to help them increase their independence.

Grading the Activity
Directions: Describe ways you might grade this activity in terms of:

1. Duration/endurance
   Have more than one pair of socks to clean. Give longer time limits for rubbing the socks together or rinsing them underwater
2. Range of motion
   Change the position of the body in relation to the sink. Reaching for the soap or the socks. Changing where the washboard is set up, its height and angle
3. Resistance
   Put weights on the person's wrists. Use socks that are made out of heavier yarn so that they do not slide past each other as easily upon rubbing
4. Complexity
   Structuring the task for different colors of socks, and different textures of socks (some are considered delicate; need to identify the socks that should be rubbed gently)
5. Independence
   A person who is functioning at a low cognitive ability may need some assistance at first

Form 3-2a.
PATIENT-ACTIVITY CORRELATION FORM

Student: _Example (based on Profile 2 - Mary and Joe Wells)_

Course: _____ Date: _____

1. Patient Profile
   Mary and Joe are young married adults with spastic cerebral palsy. Both are wheelchair-bound. They have been referred to occupational therapy for the independent management of their clothing during a vacation.

2. Therapeutic Goals
   a. Long-term
   The patients will reach independence in the selection and care of their lightweight clothing.

   b. Short-term
   The patients will wash their socks in the bathroom sink, in regard to the independence of the management of their clothing.

3. Goal-Directed Activity Description
   The patients will gather together all materials needed to wash their socks, and organize them at the bathroom sink. They will then proceed to wash, rinse, and dry the socks for the purpose of learning to independently care for their clothing.

4. Activity Preparation Requirements
   a. Task
   N/A

   b. Personnel
   One therapist will be needed to supervise the activity.

   c. Preparation time
   Preparation will take about 2 min. to gather and organize the materials needed for the activity.

   d. Place/space
   Enough room is needed near the sink in the bathroom so that the patients can maneuver their wheelchairs without difficulty.

   e. Materials
   N/A

   f. Equipment
   N/A

   g. Safety precautions (personnel)
   N/A

Form 3-2a. (continued)

5. Activity Implementation Requirements
   a. Personnel
      N/A

   b. Setting/location
      N/A

   c. Area/space
      Enough room is needed in the bathroom near the sink so that the patients can maneuver their wheelchairs without difficulty.

   d. Environment
      No special environment is needed in the bathroom to perform this activity.

   e. Materials
      N/A

   f. Equipment/adaptations
      Equipment needed includes the sink, faucet, soap, water, and socks.

   g. Time frame
      N/A

   h. Safety precautions (patient)
      The water temperature should be comfortable to touch, and rubber gloves can be used for protection against possible soap irritation and bumping of the knuckles.

6. Activity Sequence (Action steps: ten or less)
   a. *Gather and organize all the materials needed for washing the socks*
   b. *Fill the plugged sink with soap and water*
   c. *Begin washing the socks needed for appropriate dressing*
   d. *After they are clean, rinse and wring the water from the socks*
   e. *Hang the socks over the sink edge until they are dry enough to wear*

7. Therapeutic Application
   INDEPENDENT LIVING/DAILY LIVING SKILLS
      Physical daily living skills
         Grooming and hygiene
         Dressing
         Functional mobility
         Object manipulation
      Psychological/emotional daily living skills
         Situational coping
   PSYCHOSOCIAL COMPONENTS
      Self-management
         Self-control

Form 3-3.
ACTIVITY ANALYSIS FORM

Student: _Example_   Date: _____

Course: _____

Part I - Activity Summary
Directions: Respond to the following in list format.

1. Name of activity
   Painting a bedroom wall

2. Brief description of activity
   The student will evenly distribute paint to the bedroom wall with a roller and brush

3. Tools/equipment (nonexpendable), cost and source
   Roller—$3, hardware store; paint pan—$2, hardware store; step ladder—$35, hardware store; paint brush—$5, hardware store

4. Materials/supplies (expendable), cost and source
   One gallon of paint—$16, hardware store; paint roller covers—$2, hardware store; soap—$.59, grocery store; masking tape—$5, hardware store; newspaper— free, home

5. Space/environmental requirements
   Remove furniture from the bedroom and open window for ventilation. Clean the wall of debris, place newspaper on floor, and put masking tape on the baseboards

6. Sequence of major steps; time required for each step
   a. *Pour paint into pan carefully: 30 sec.*
   b. *Place lid on can tightly: 45 sec.*
   c. *Put roller cover on securely: 1 min.*
   d. *Distribute paint on roller evenly: 30 sec.*
   e. *Use vertical strokes to paint wall repeatedly: 1-2 min. for each stroke*
   f. *Dip roller intermittently: 2 min.*
   g. *Dip paint brush into pan carefully: 30 sec.*
   h. *Apply paint to trim horizontally with brush: 15 min.*
   i. *Clean brush with soap thoroughly: 2 min.*
   j. *Let paint dry evenly: 2 hrs.*

7. Precautions (review "Sequence of major steps")
   The ladder will be stable. The room will be well ventilated to avoid fumes. The student will use proper body mechanics when removing the furniture to avoid muscle strain. The student will be cautious when pouring the paint to eliminate spills. The student will place lid on paint can tightly to assure that the paint will not evaporate.

8. Contraindications (review participant's status)
   No contradictions with student as participant

9. Special considerations (age appropriateness, educational requirements, cultural relevance, sexual identification, other)
   No special considerations apply with student as participant

10. Acceptable criteria for completed project
    An evenly painted bedroom wall with no drips or uncovered blemishes. It should have a smooth finish with no holes

Form 3-3. (continued)

Part II - Occupational Performance Components

Directions: Indicate the skill components necessary to complete the task (as it is normally done). State your reasoning to the right of each item. Write "N/A" if not applicable. Refer to Uniform Terminology (Appendix B) for definitions of terms.

A. Sensorimotor Components
1. Neuromuscular
   a. Reflex integration
      Necessary to allow voluntary movement
   b. Range of motion
      (1) active
         Upper extremity involvement is necessary to apply the paint. The patient uses full joint movement
      (2) passive
         N/A
      (3) active assistive
         N/A
   c. Gross and fine coordination
      (1) muscle control
         Necessary to direct movements to paint the wall
      (2) coordination
         Must have controlled movement of back, legs, arms, and pectoral muscles to complete the task
      (3) dexterity
         Need to use small muscle groups, such as those in the hand, to hold the paint brush
   d. Strength and endurance
      (1) building strength, cardiopulmonary reserve
         N/A
      (2) increasing length of work period
         N/A
      (3) decreasing fatigue/strain
         Strain results from using infrequently used muscles excessively
2. Sensory integration
   a. Sensory awareness
      (1) tactile awareness
         Needed to perceive that he or she is holding a brush or roller
      (2) stereognosis
         N/A
      (3) kinesthesia
         Consciously perceiving motion, weight, and position of arm while applying paint
      (4) proprioceptive awareness
         Need to be aware of the position of body in space
      (5) ocular control
         Use visual tracking of the paint roller
      (6) vestibular awareness
         Necessary to detect motion and gravity and to keep her balance while painting
      (7) auditory awareness
         N/A
      (8) gustatory awareness
         N/A

Form 3-3. (continued)

      (9) olfactory awareness
          Awareness of the paint's odor
   b. Visual-spatial awareness
      (1) figure-ground
          Needed to be able to distinguish the painted parts from the nonpainted
      (2) form constancy
          N/A
      (3) position in space
          Needed to be aware of body in relation to the wall, ladder, and floor
   c. Body integration
      (1) body schema
          Awareness of the position of body and sore muscles
      (2) postural balance
          Necessary to maintain posture and balance while painting on a ladder
      (3) bilateral motor coordination
          Used when the student pours the paint into the pan
      (4) right-left discrimination
          N/A
      (5) visual-motor integration
          Hand-eye coordination is needed to paint the wall
      (6) crossing the midline
          Depending on the position of the body in relation to the wall, crossing the midline may occur
      (7) praxis
          Must develop a plan of how to grasp the roller and paint the wall

B. Cognitive Components
   1. Orientation
     Need to be aware of appropriate clothing for the task
   2. Conceptualization/comprehension
     a. Concentration
       Necessary to focus on a goal
     b. Attention span
       Must focus on painting until the task was finished
     c. Memory
       Long-term memory was used to recall how to paint, and short-term memory was used to remember where tools are
   3. Cognitive integration
     a. Generalization
       The student uses general knowledge of painting to facilitate the painting of this wall
     b. Problem solving
      (1) defining or evaluating the problem
          Need to realize the wall needs to be painted
      (2) organizing a plan
          Must know what tools were needed and how the process could be accomplished
      (3) making decisions/judgment
          Need to decide which tools and what color paint to purchase
      (4) implementing a plan
          Must buy the tools and paint the wall

Form 3-3. (continued)

(5) evaluating decision/judgment

After completing the task, the student evaluates the job she has done

C. Psychosocial Components
   1. Self-management
      a. Self-expression
         (1) experiencing/recognizing a range of emotions

         The student may get frustrated if the task is not going as planned, and the student may experience joy when the job is finished

         (2) having an adequate vocabulary

         N/A

         (3) writing and speaking skills

         N/A

         (4) use of nonverbal signs and symbols

         N/A

      b. Self-control
         (1) observing own and others' behavior

         The student observes own behavior

         (2) recognizing need for behavior/action change

         The student realizes, when frustrated, that a mood change is necessary for a better end product

         (3) imitating new behaviors

         N/A

         (4) directing energies into stress-reducing behaviors

         N/A

   2. Dyadic interaction
      a. Understanding norms of communication and interaction

      N/A

      b. Setting limits on self and others

      The student decided not to quit until the task was complete

      c. Compromising and negotiating

      N/A

      d. Handling stress

      The student needs to overcome stress to work efficiently

      e. Cooperating and competing with others

      N/A

      f. Responsibly relying on self and others

      The student relies on self to complete the task

   3. Group interaction
      a. Performing social/emotional roles and tasks

      N/A

      b. Understanding simple group process

      N/A

      c. Participating in a mutually beneficial group

      N/A

Form 3-3. (continued)

D. Task Requirements
1. Work patterns
   a. Light
   N/A

   b. Moderate
   The student is not aerobically involved but is using some major muscle groups

   c. Heavy
   N/A

2. Method
   a. Structured
   N/A

   b. Methodical
   Painting the wall has an orderly arrangement in that the student puts one stroke of paint right next to the last

   c. Repetitive
   The stroking of the paint onto the wall is done repeatedly

   d. Expressive
   N/A

   e. Creative
   N/A

   f. Orderly
   Needed in order not to spill the paint

   g. Physical contact
   The student comes into contact with the roller, brush, paint can and pan

   h. Projective
   N/A

Form 3-3. (continued)

Part III - Occupational Performance
Directions: Indicate possible treatment goals that this activity might address in one or more of the areas of occupational performance. State your reasoning as in Part I. Write "N/A" if not applicable.

A. Independent Living/Daily Living Skills
   1. Physical daily living skills
      a. Grooming and hygiene
         N/A
      b. Feeding/eating
         N/A
      c. Dressing
         N/A
      d. Functional mobility
         N/A
      e. Functional communication
         N/A
      f. Object manipulation
         Used to handle the paint brush and roller

   2. Psychological/emotional daily living skills
      a. Self-concept/self-identity
         N/A
      b. Situational coping
         The student initiated, implemented, and followed through on the decision to paint the wall
      c. Community involvement
         N/A

   3. Work
      a. Homemaking
         Painting the wall prepares the student's home to be a pleasing living environment
      b. Child care/parenting
         N/A
      c. Employment preparation
         N/A

   4. Play/leisure
      a. Recognizing one's needs
         N/A
      b. Identifying characteristics of play
         N/A
      c. Selecting play activities
         N/A
      d. Adaptation of activities
         N/A
      e. Utilizing community resources
         N/A

Form 3-3. (continued)

Part IV - Occupational Performance Modifications
Directions: Indicate ways this activity might be modified to increase independent function. State your reasoning. Write "N/A" if not applicable.

Note: This activity should be done with the non-dominant hand only.

A. Therapeutic Adaptation
  1. Orthotics
    a. Static or dynamic positioning
      N/A
    b. Relieve pain
      N/A
    c. Maintain joint alignment
      N/A
    d. Protect joint integrity
      N/A
    e. Improve function
      N/A
    f. Decrease deformity
      N/A

  2. Prosthetics
    N/A

  3. Assistive/adaptive equipment
    a. Architectural modification
      N/A
    b. Environmental modification
      A paint pan that is larger may be necessary to catch drips and spills that are due to uncoordinated activity
    c. Assistive equipment
      Longer handled paint roller, something under wrist for extra support
    d. Wheelchair modification
      N/A

B. Prevention
  1. Energy conservation
    a. Energy-saving procedures
      Using a longer handle on roller
    b. Activity restriction
      N/A
    c. Work simplification
      Use a cup to get paint from can to tray
    d. Time management
      Allowing more time because the task would not be performed as easily
    e. Environmental organization
      Keeping window open for ventilation

Form 3-3. (continued)

2. Joint protection/body mechanics
   a. Proper body mechanics
      Bending at the knees instead of at the back
   b. Avoiding static/deforming postures
      Move entire body not just arm
   c. Avoiding excessive weight bearing
      N/A
   d. Positioning
      Painting the portion that is directly in front of body
   e. Coordinating daily living activities
      N/A

Implications for Treatment
Directions: Explain how and for whom this activity could be beneficial. Indicate physical and/or psychosocial dysfunction.

Physical: Increased shoulder strength and motion are gained; eye-hand coordination is worked on.

Psychosocial: Self-control is required to get the wall painted; painting the wall would be accomplishing a goal (increased self-esteem).

Grading the Activity
Directions: Describe ways you might grade this activity in terms of:

1. Duration/endurance
   Work for longer periods without a break

2. Range of motion
   Working without a ladder would increase joint movement

3. Resistance
   Place weights on wrists

4. Complexity
   Use brush for entire wall instead of roller

5. Independence
   Obtain all materials without assistance

Form 3-3a.
PATIENT-ACTIVITY CORRELATION FORM

Student: _Example (based on Profile 3 — Wendy Jenkins)_

Course: _____ Date: _____

1. Patient Profile

    Patient is a 15-year-old female student suffering from Oppositional Defiance Disorder. Her symptoms include being openly defiant with her parents and teachers. She states that her parents/teachers will not allow her to express her feelings and that they "boss" her too much. The referral to occupational therapy was made for an assessment and treatment in terms of activities that will permit the patient to have control with specific areas of space/time without adult supervision.

2. Therapeutic Goals

    a. Long-Term

    Patient will develop appropriate situational behavior with her parents and teachers.

    b. Short-Term

    Patient will achieve independence through self-expression and responsibility with set guidelines.

3. Goal-Directed Activity Description

    The patient will paint her bedroom wall. She will determine the materials needed and purchase the materials with guidance from her parents. Grading of the activity will occur at different times to increase her tolerance of authority figures and to elicit proper self-expression.

4. Activity Preparation Requirements

    a. Task

    _N/A_

    b. Personnel

    An occupational therapist to supervise the activity

    c. Preparation time

    Approximately 30 min. to discuss with patient and parents what needs to be accomplished

    d. Place/space

    An empty bedroom

    e. Materials

    _N/A_

    f. Equipment

    _N/A_

    g. Safety precautions (personnel)

    _N/A_

5. Activity Implementation Requirements

    a. Personnel

    _N/A_

    b. Setting/location

    _N/A_

Form 3-3a. (continued)

c. **Area/space**
Empty bedroom

d. **Environment**
No parent intervention except for praise

e. **Materials**
N/A

f. **Equipment/adaptations**
Roller pan, ladder, paint brush, paint, roller brush covers, soap, masking tape, newspaper.

g. **Time frame**
N/A

h. **Safety precautions (patient)**
If patient becomes frustrated, stop the activity to allow for self-expression through discussion with therapist so that anger doesn't occur and present problems.

6. **Activity Sequence (Action steps: ten or less)**
   a. *Go to hardware store to purchase materials with minimal guidance from parents*
   b. *Organize environment carefully*
   c. *Organize materials in room functionally*
   d. *Paint her bedroom wall with expression of self*
   e. *Evaluate work objectively*
   f. *Clean any messes independently.*

7. **Therapeutic Application**
INDEPENDENT LIVING/DAILY LIVING SKILLS
  Psychological/emotional daily living skills
    Self-concept/self-identity
      realistically perceiving others' needs, feelings, conflicts, values, expectations
      sensing one's competence, achievement, self-esteem, and self-respect
      integrating new experiences with established self-concept/self-identity
    Situational coping
      perceiving changes and need for changes in self and environment
      directing and redirecting energy to overcome problems
      assuming responsibility for self and consequences of actions
      interacting with others, dyadic, and group
COGNITIVE COMPONENTS
  Cognitive integration
    Problem solving
PSYCHOSOCIAL COMPONENTS
  Self-management
    Self-expression
      experiencing and recognizing a range of emotions
    Self-control
      conceptualizing problems in terms of needed behavioral changes or actions
      directing and redirecting energies into stress-reducing activities and behaviors
  Dyadic interaction
    Compromising and negotiating
    Handling competition, frustration, anxiety, success, and failure
    Cooperating and competing with others

Form 3-4.
ACTIVITY ANALYSIS FORM

Student: _Example_ _____ Date: _____
Course: _____

Part I - Activity Summary
Directions: Respond to the following in list format.

1. Name of activity
   Washing dishes in the sink

2. Brief description of activity
   The student will pile dishes into sink of soapy water, scrub with sponge, rinse with water, and set on rack to dry.

3. Tools/equipment (nonexpendable), cost and source
   Sink—$40, hardware store; dishes—$30, department store; sponge—$1, department store; drying rack—$5, department store

4. Materials/supplies (expendable), cost and source
   Water—free, included in rent, from utility company; soap—$2, grocery store

5. Space/environmental requirements
   Kitchen with enough room to stand/sit and manipulate objects in front of sink is needed. Countertop with enough room to place drying rack is needed. No specific environmental requirements.

6. Sequence of major steps; time required for each step
   a. Fill empty sink with warm water: 2 min.
   b. Add small amount of soap to water, allowing suds to form: 5 sec.
   c. Place dirty dishes in water: 1 min.
   d. Scrub each dish individually: 10 min.
   e. Rinse each dish individually: 5 min.
   f. Place clean dish on rack to dry: 3 min.

7. Precautions (review "Sequence of major steps")
   Handle the dishes carefully, especially sharp objects, and make sure the water temperature is tolerable to the skin.

8. Contraindications (review participant's status)
   N/A

9. Special considerations (age appropriateness, educational requirements, cultural relevance, sexual identification, other)
   N/A

10. Acceptable criteria for completed project
    Clean and rinsed dishes

Form 3-4. (continued)

Part II - Occupational Performance Components
Directions: Indicate the skill components necessary to complete the task (as it is normally done). State your reasoning to the right of each item. Write "N/A" if not applicable. Refer to Uniform Terminology (Appendix B) for definitions of terms.

A. Sensorimotor Components
   1. Neuromuscular
      a. Reflex integration
         Reflexes need to be integrated for smooth, coordinated, voluntary movement
      b. Range of motion
         (1) active
            Necessary to perform movements and manipulate objects (washing dishes, moving to drying rack)
         (2) passive
            N/A
         (3) active assistive
            N/A
      c. Gross and fine coordination
         (1) muscle control
            Necessary to coordinate and direct movement
         (2) coordination
            Necessary for gross and fine motor control
         (3) dexterity
            Necessary for fine movements used for grasping small objects and sponge
      d. Strength and endurance
         (1) building strength, cardiopulmonary reserve
            N/A
         (2) increasing length of work period
            N/A
         (3) decreasing fatigue/strain
            N/A
   2. Sensory integration
      a. Sensory awareness
         (1) tactile awareness
            Necessary for testing water temperature
         (2) stereognosis
            Necessary for identifying and discriminating unseen objects under surface of water
         (3) kinesthesia
            Necessary for awareness of hand movements in relation to objects and sink
         (4) proprioceptive awareness
            Necessary for awareness of hand and body position in relation to objects and sink
         (5) ocular control
            Necessary to visually locate objects used in washing dishes
         (6) vestibular awareness
            Necessary to maintain balance and posture while standing at the sink
         (7) auditory awareness
            N/A
         (8) gustatory awareness
            N/A

Form 3-4. (continued)

       (9) olfactory awareness
          N/A
    b. Visual-spatial awareness
       (1) figure ground
          Necessary to distinguish particular dishes from others and from the water
       (2) form constancy
          N/A
       (3) position in space
          Necessary to be aware of body parts in relation to sink and space around it
    c. Body integration
       (1) body schema
          Necessary to recognize the physical self in reference to the task
       (2) postural balance
          Necessary to maintain balance and posture while standing at sink
       (3) bilateral motor coordination
          Necessary to coordinate holding and washing movements between both hands
       (4) right-left discrimination
          N/A
       (5) visual-motor integration
          Hand-eye coordination is necessary to manipulate dishes smoothly and effectively
       (6) crossing the midline
          Necessary to grasp and watch objects that are lateral to midline as well as directly in front
       (7) praxis
          Necessary for planning coordinated movement of dishes

B. Cognitive Components
  1. Orientation
     Necessary to know what the task is (washing dishes)
  2. Conceptualization/comprehension
    a. Concentration
       N/A
    b. Attention span
       Necessary to focus on completion of washing all dishes
    c. Memory
       Necessary to remember how to wash dishes
  3. Cognitive integration
    a. Generalization
       Can be applied to washing other objects in the sink
    b. Problem solving
       (1) defining or evaluating the problem
          Must realize dishes need to be washed
       (2) organizing a plan
          Must decide steps to follow in washing dishes
       (3) making decisions/judgment
          Must decide how clean is "clean enough"
       (4) implementing a plan
          Must follow through with previously organized plan
       (5) evaluating decision/judgment
          Must decide if the dishes are, in fact, clean

Form 3-4. (continued)

C. Psychosocial Components
1. Self-management
    a. Self-expression
        (1) experiencing/recognizing a range of emotions
            N/A
        (2) having an adequate vocabulary
            N/A
        (3) writing and speaking skills
            N/A
        (4) use of nonverbal signs and symbols
            N/A
    b. Self-control
        (1) observing own and others' behaviors
            N/A
        (2) recognizing need for behavior/action change
            N/A
        (3) imitating new behaviors
            N/A
        (4) directing energy into stress-reducing behaviors
            N/A

2. Dyadic interaction
    a. Understanding norms of communication and interaction
        N/A
    b. Setting limits on self and others
        N/A
    c. Compromising and negotiating
        N/A
    d. Handling stress
        N/A
    e. Cooperating and competing with others
        N/A
    f. Responsibly relying on self and others
        N/A

3. Group interaction
    a. Performing social/emotional roles and tasks
        N/A
    b. Understanding simple group process
        N/A
    c. Participating in a mutually beneficial group
        N/A

Form 3-4. (continued)

D. Task Requirements
   1. Work patterns
      a. Light
         Minimal physical work is required

      b. Moderate
         N/A

      c. Heavy
         N/A

   2. Method
      a. Structured
         Follow a set plan

      b. Methodical
         Follow a set sequence

      c. Repetitive
         Follow a set sequence a number of times

      d. Expressive
         N/A

      e. Creative
         N/A

      f. Orderly
         Must make sure dishes are thoroughly cleaned and make sure to not make a mess with soap and water

      g. Physical contact
         N/A

      h. Projective
         N/A

Form 3-4. (continued)

Part III - Occupational Performance

Directions: Indicate possible treatment goals that this activity might address in one or more of the areas of occupational performance. State your reasoning as in Part I. Write "N/A" if not applicable.

A. Independent Living/Daily Living Skills
   1. Physical daily living skills
      a. Grooming and hygiene
         N/A
      b. Feeding/eating
         N/A
      c. Dressing
         N/A
      d. Functional mobility
         N/A
      e. Functional communication
         N/A
      f. Object manipulation
         Handling and washing dishes is a daily task a homemaker must fulfill

   2. Psychological/emotional daily living skills
      a. Self-concept/self-identity
         N/A
      b. Situational coping
         N/A
      c. Community involvement
         N/A

   3. Work
      a. Homemaking
         Washing dishes is a task a homemaker does
      b. Child care/parenting
         N/A
      c. Employment preparation
         N/A

   4. Play/leisure
      a. Recognizing one's needs
         N/A
      b. Identifying characteristics of play
         N/A
      c. Selecting play activities
         N/A
      d. Adaptation of activities
         N/A
      e. Utilizing community resources
         N/A

Form 3-4. (continued)

Part IV - Occupational Performance Modifications
Directions: Indicate ways this activity might be modified to increase independent function. State your reasoning. Write "N/A" if not applicable.

Note: This activity should be done with the non-dominant hand only.

A. Therapeutic Adaptations
   1. Orthotics
      a. Static or dynamic positioning
        N/A
      b. Relieve pain
        N/A
      c. Maintain joint alignment
        N/A
      d. Protect joint integrity
        N/A
      e. Improve function
        N/A
      f. Decrease deformity
        N/A

   2. Prosthetics
   N/A

   3. Assistive/adaptive equipment
      a. Architectural modification
        N/A
      b. Environmental modification
        Move drying rack to left side of sink. Put soapy water in right side, rinse water in left side
      c. Assistive equipment
        Place a sheet of "dycem" on right counter top to hold dishes in place while washing with left hand
      d. Wheelchair modification
        N/A

B. Prevention
   1. Energy conservation
      a. Energy-saving procedures
        Moving in a sequence from right to left (instead of left to right)
      b. Activity restriction
        N/A
      c. Work simplification
        Using dycem to hold objects in place while washing simplifies job. Bottle brush makes washing glasses simpler
      d. Time management
        Using the right to left system in an orderly fashion to efficiently wash the dishes
      e. Environmental organization
        Organizing the process from right to left facilitates the dishwashing process

Form 3-4. (continued)

2. Joint protection/body mechanics
   a. Proper body mechanics
      N/A
   b. Avoiding static/deforming postures
      N/A
   c. Avoiding excessive weight bearing
      N/A
   d. Positioning
      Will need to shift weight and step to the side slightly in order to easily reach all work areas
   e. Coordinating daily living activities
      N/A

Implications for Treatment
Directions: Explain how and for whom this activity could be beneficial. Indicate physical and/or psychosocial dysfunction.

Physical: Use for people with physical dysfunction: upper extremity amputee, stroke, people with decreased endurance, hip/leg rehab, people with decreased coordination (Parkinson's).

Psychosocial: Use with patients with attention-span deficits, problem-solving deficits, confidence deficits.

Grading the Activity
Directions: Describe the ways you might grade this activity in terms of:

1. Duration/endurance
   Increase or decrease the load of dishes
2. Range of motion
   N/A
3. Resistance
   Use heavier dishes, use weights on wrists, make dishes dirtier (need more intense scrubbing)
4. Complexity
   Vary the shape, size, and weight of dishes. Add steps to make the activity more complex (clear table, dry, and put away dishes)
5. Independence
   Use appropriate adaptive equipment to promote independent functioning

Form 3-4a.
PATIENT-ACTIVITY CORRELATION FORM

Student: _Example (based on Profile 4 — Alice Murphy)_

Course: _____ Date: _____

1. Patient Profile

   Patient (Alice Murphy) is a 47-year-old female with rheumatoid arthritis throughout her upper extremities. She also experiences pain and stiffness in her knees in the morning causing home management to be difficult. The patient has been referred to occupational therapy for homemaking skills, joint protection, and energy conservation.

2. Therapeutic Goals
   a. Long-term

      Patient will achieve maximum independence in homemaking and home management skills with minimal arthritic pain.

   b. Short-term

      In view of the long-term goal, the patient will wash dishes independently using adaptive equipment for joint protection and energy conservation.

3. Goal-Directed Activity Description

   Patient will wash dishes using a wash mitt to keep hand extended and also dycem to hold dishes in place. She also will sit on a tall stool or chair for decreasing pain in knees and for conserving energy.

4. Activity Preparation Requirements
   a. Task

      _N/A_

   b. Personnel

      One occupational therapist for supervising

   c. Preparation time

      The therapist will take 2-3 min. to get the stool, dycem, and wash mitt ready to use at the sink.

   d. Place/space

      Space behind the kitchen sink and the surrounding countertop in the occupational therapy clinic

   e. Materials

      _N/A_

   f. Equipment

      _N/A_

   g. Safety precautions (personnel)

      _N/A_

Form 3-4a. (continued)

5. Activity Implementation Requirements
   a. Personnel
      N/A
   b. Setting/location
      N/A
   c. Area/space
      Space behind the sink and the nearby countertop for the drying rack
   d. Environment
      Kitchen in occupational therapy clinic
   e. Materials
      N/A
   f. Equipment/adaptations
      Dycem, wash mitt, stool, sink, water, dish liquid, drying rack, and utensils or dishes
   g. Time frame
      N/A
   h. Safety precautions (patient)
      The stool should be sturdy and supportive to avoid injury, the water should be lukewarm in temperature, and breakable dishes and knives should be handled carefully.

6. Activity Sequence (Action steps: ten or less)
   a. *Patient will position self on stool carefully to relieve joint pain and stiffness.*
   b. *Patient will fill the sink with soap and warm water which will sooth arthritic pain and facilitate mobility.*
   c. *Patient will fill the other side of the sink with warm water for rinsing dishes to cut down on excessive movement.*
   d. *Patient will place the dirty dishes in the soapy water using joint protection techniques.*
   e. *Patient will place each dirty dish on dycem and scrub with the mitt to keep fingers extended while using joint protection techniques.*
   f. *Using bilateral motor coordination, the patient will pick up the clean dish with the left hand and place it in the clean, rinsing water.*
   g. *The patient will place each clean dish in the drying rack.*

7. Therapeutic Application
   INDEPENDENT LIVING/DAILY LIVING SKILLS
   Work
   Homemaking
   SENSORIMOTOR COMPONENTS
   Neuromuscular
   Range of motion
   active
   Strength and endurance
   THERAPEUTIC ADAPTATIONS
   Assistive/adaptive equipment
   Dycem
   Wash mitt
   Tall stool
   PREVENTION
   Energy conservation
   Joint protection/body mechanics
   Positioning

Form 3-5.
ACTIVITY ANALYSIS FORM

Student: _Example_ _____ Date: _____

Course: _____

Part I - Activity Summary
Directions: Respond to the following in list format.

1. Name of activity
   Making a turkey sandwich

2. Brief description of activity
   The student will place turkey with desired condiments between two pieces of bread.

3. Tools/equipment (nonexpendable), cost and source
   Knife—$1, general

4. Material/supplies (expendable), cost and source
   Bread (two slices)—$.10, Krogers; turkey, 1/8 lb.—$.50, Krogers; cheese (one slice)—$.10, Krogers; mayonnaise, 1 T—$.01, Krogers

5. Space/environmental requirements
   A 2 ft. × 2 ft. kitchen counter area is needed to perform the task. Refrigeration is needed for materials.

6. Sequence of major steps; time required for each step
   a. _Place all necessary items on counter carefully: 20 sec._
   b. _Spread mayonnaise on both slices of bread equally: 6 sec._
   c. _Place slices of turkey on one slice of bread neatly: 3 sec._
   d. _Position cheese on bread proportionately: 3 sec._
   e. _Place second slice of bread on cheese successfully: 1 sec._

7. Precautions (review "Sequence of major steps")
   Keep the work area clean to avoid food contamination and clean up any spills immediately. Use a dull blunt knife to avoid accidents and use nonbreakable containers for condiments.

8. Contraindications (review participant's status)
   None

9. Special considerations (age appropriateness, educational requirements, cultural relevance, sexual identification, other)
   Appropriate for college level person

10. Acceptable criteria for completed project
    A turkey sandwich that is pleasing to the eye, satisfying to the taste buds, and nutritious for the body

Form 3-5. (continued)

Part II - Occupational Performance Components
Directions: Indicate the skill components necessary to complete the task (as it is normally done). State your reasoning to the right of each item. Write "N/A" if not applicable.

A. Sensorimotor Components
  1. Neuromuscular
    a. Reflex integration
      Needed for voluntary movement
    b. Range of motion
      (1) active
        Activity is done independently
      (2) passive
        N/A
      (3) active assistive
        N/A
    c. Gross and fine coordination
      (1) muscle control
        Needed to direct muscles in hands and arms while making the turkey sandwich
      (2) coordination
        Needed for gross motor movement of arms to position food materials
      (3) dexterity
        Needed for fine movements of wrists and fingers while preparing sandwich
    d. Strength and endurance
      (1) building strength, cardiopulmonary reserve
        N/A
      (2) increasing length of work period
        N/A
      (3) decreasing fatigue/strain
        N/A
  2. Sensory integration
    a. Sensory awareness
      (1) tactile awareness
        Needed to distinguish between ingredients used to make the sandwich
      (2) stereognosis
        N/A
      (3) kinesthesia
        Necessary for positioning of body during process
      (4) proprioception awareness
        Needed for identification of body position while sitting or standing
      (5) ocular control
        Needed to see materials
      (6) vestibular awareness
        Needed to maintain position and balance while working
      (7) auditory awareness
        N/A
      (8) gustatory awareness
        Needed to taste food
      (9) olfactory awareness
        Necessary to smell for spoilage of ingredients

Form 3-5. (continued)

   b. Visual-spatial awareness
   - (1) figure-ground
     N/A
   - (2) form constancy
     N/A
   - (3) position in space
     Necessary to know where body is in relationship to materials
   c. Body integration
   - (1) body schema
     Perception of position and action of all body parts during activity
   - (2) postural balance
     Needed to stand or sit at work place
   - (3) bilateral motor coordination
     Needed to hold bread with one hand while using the other hand to spread mayonnaise on bread
   - (4) right-left discrimination
     N/A
   - (5) visual-motor integration
     Need hand-eye coordination in putting sandwich together
   - (6) crossing the midline
     Needed to use arm in swiping motion while spreading mayonnaise on bread
   - (7) praxis
     Needed to plan steps of making the turkey sandwich

B. Cognitive Components
   1. Orientation
      Needed to identify place and situation while performing task
   2. Conceptualization/comprehension
      a. Concentration
         Must be able to concentrate long enough to complete the task
      b. Attention span
         Requires less than 1 min.
      c. Memory
         Must be able to remember steps involved in making the turkey sandwich
   3. Cognitive integration
      a. Generalization
         Previous concept of preparing a sandwich could be applied
      b. Problem solving
      - (1) defining or evaluating the problem
        Used to decide how the sandwich will be made and what ingredients are needed
      - (2) organizing a plan
        Needed to gather appropriate materials
      - (3) making decisions/judgment
        Making decisions on the amount of ingredients to be put on sandwich
      - (4) implementing a plan
        The actual process of making the turkey sandwich
      - (5) evaluating decision/judgment
        To determine, by appearance and taste, if you want to add anything else to sandwich

Form 3-5. (continued)

C. Psychosocial Components
  1. Self-management
    a. Self-expression
      (1) experiencing/recognizing a range of emotions
          N/A
      (2) having an adequate vocabulary
          N/A
      (3) writing and speaking skills
          N/A
      (4) use of non-verbal signs and symbols
          N/A
    b. Self-control
      (1) observing own and others' behavior
          N/A
      (2) recognizing need for behavior/action change
          N/A
      (3) imitating new behaviors
          N/A
      (4) directing energies into stress-reducing behaviors
          N/A

  2. Dyadic interaction
    a. Understanding norms of communication and interaction
       N/A
    b. Setting limits on self and others
       N/A
    c. Compromising and negotiating
       N/A
    d. Handling stress
       N/A
    e. Cooperating and competing with others
       N/A
    f. Responsibly relying on self and others
       N/A

  3. Group interaction
    a. Performing social/emotional roles and tasks
       N/A
    b. Understanding simple group process
       N/A
    c. Participating in a mutually beneficial group
       N/A

Form 3-5. (continued)

D. Task Requirements
   1. Work patterns
      a. Light
         No heavy physical labor required

      b. Moderate
         N/A

      c. Heavy
         N/A

   2. Method
      a. Structured
         There are elements (bread, filling, etc.) that define the structure which equals a sandwich

      b. Methodical
         Certain sequence of steps followed

      c. Repetitive
         N/A

      d. Expressive
         N/A

      e. Creative
         Task allows person to be creative and to add ingredients that they would like to eat on sandwich

      f. Orderly
         Necessary to have a noncontaminated sandwich

      g. Physical contact
         N/A

      h. Projective
         N/A

Form 3-5. (continued)

Part III - Occupational Performance
Directions: Indicate possible treatment goals that this activity might address in one or more of the areas of occupational performance. State your reasoning as in Part I. Write "N/A" if not applicable.

A. Independent Living/Daily Living Skills
  1. Physical daily living skills
    a. Grooming and hygiene
      Important in meal preparation
    b. Feeding/eating
      Essential for meal preparation
    c. Dressing
      N/A
    d. Functional mobility
      Being able to move about kitchen
    e. Functional communication
      N/A
    f. Object manipulation
      Working with utensils and materials

  2. Psychological/emotional daily living skills
    a. Self-concept/self-identity
      Motivation and satisfaction of performing task
    b. Situational coping
      Coping using nondominant hand or adaptive equipment
    c. Community involvement
      N/A

  3. Work
    a. Homemaking
      N/A
    b. Child care/parenting
      N/A
    c. Employment preparation
      N/A

  4. Play/leisure
    a. Recognizing one's needs
      N/A
    b. Identifying characteristics of play
      N/A
    c. Selecting play activities
      N/A
    d. Adaptation of activities
      N/A
    e. Utilizing community resources
      N/A

Form 3-5. (continued)

Part IV - Occupational Performance Modifications
Directions: Indicate ways this activity might be modified to increase independent function.
State your reasoning. Write "N/A" if not applicable.

Note: This activity should be done with the non-dominant hand only.

A. Therapeutic Adaptations
   1. Orthotics
      a. Static or dynamic positioning
         N/A
      b. Relieve pain
         N/A
      c. Maintain joint alignment
         N/A
      d. Protect joint integrity
         N/A
      e. Improve function
         N/A
      f. Decrease deformity
         N/A

   2. Prosthetics
      N/A

   3. Assistive/adaptive equipment
      a. Architectural modification
         N/A
      b. Environmental modification
         N/A
      c. Assistive equipment
         Cutting board
      d. Wheelchair modification
         N/A

B. Prevention
   1. Energy conservation
      a. Energy-saving procedures
         N/A
      b. Activity restriction
         N/A
      c. Work simplification
         N/A
      d. Time management
         N/A
      e. Environmental organization
         N/A

Form 3-5. (continued)

2. Joint protection/body mechanics
   a. Proper body mechanics
      N/A
   b. Avoiding static/deforming postures
      Alter body positions as needed
   c. Avoiding excessive weight bearing
      N/A
   d. Positioning
      Modify posture
   e. Coordinating daily living activities
      Food preparation involves components of daily living skills that can help achieve different treatment goals.

Implications for Treatment

Directions: Explain how and for whom this activity could be beneficial. Indicate physical and/or psychosocial dysfunction.

Physical: This activity would be useful for upper extremity disabilities. A stroke patient who has lost the use of his dominant hand would regain strength and mobility. An amputee who has lost a dominant hand would learn to perform task with nondominant hand or with artificial hand. This activity would increase mobility and strength in many upper extremity disabilities.

Psychosocial: Use as a model for daily living skills with psychosocial dysfunctions. Patients with dependent personalities would increase independence by making their own meals. A depressed patient would increase his self-esteem by successfully completing the task. A patient with anorexia nervosa would be encouraged to deal with food and food preparation.

Grading the Activity

Directions: Describe ways you might grade this activity in terms of:

1. Duration/endurance
   Make one sandwich at first, then progress to making more turkey sandwiches
2. Range of motion
   Position materials differently on table
3. Resistance
   Tighten and open condiment lids
4. Complexity
   Add more ingredients and steps to follow
5. Independence
   Make decisions on what will be put on the sandwich and how the sandwich is to be made

Form 3-5a.
PATIENT-ACTIVITY CORRELATION FORM

Student: _Example (based on Profile 5 — George Handley)_

Course: _____ **Date:** _____

1. **Patient Profile**

   The patient's name is George Handley. He is a 76-year-old male. His wife died 2 months ago. He has little experience with cooking and homemaking. He visits a senior center once every day, where he gets one hot full meal at noon. He eats very little for supper. He has low motivation to eat, and as a result is noticeably thinner. Patient needs to be motivated to eat by being instructed in the importance of eating and nutrition.

2. **Therapeutic Goals**
   a. **Long-term goal**

   The patient will become proficient with independent food preparation.

   b. **Short-term goal**

   The patient will increase motivation and independence by making a turkey sandwich.

3. **Goal-Directed Activity Description**

   The client will independently select the necessary food items and prepare a turkey sandwich. He will also learn the importance of eating and nutrition.

4. **Activity Preparation Requirements**
   a. **Task**

   _N/A_

   b. **Personnel**

   Therapist only

   c. **Preparation time**

   ½ hour to be sure all necessary ingredients are available from which patient will choose

   d. **Place/space**

   Countertop and refrigerator

   e. **Materials**

   _N/A_

   f. **Equipment**

   _N/A_

   g. **Safety precautions (personnel)**

   _N/A_

Form 3-5a. (continued)

5. Activity Implementation Requirements
    a. Personnel
        N/A
    b. Setting/location
        N/A
    c. Area/space
        Countertop, minimum of 2 ft. × 2 ft.
    d. Environment
        Kitchen setting
    e. Materials
        N/A
    f. Equipment/adaptations
        Knife
    g. Time frame
        N/A
    h. Safety precautions (patient)
        Make patient knowledgeable/aware of food spoilage

6. Activity Sequence (Action steps: ten or less)
    a. The patient will select necessary food and condiment items independently.
    b. The patient will prepare a turkey sandwich as he desires triumphantly.
    c. Discuss importance of eating and nutrition sensitively.
    d. Discuss preplanning a menu and a time schedule for meals clearly.

7. Therapeutic Application
    PSYCHOSOCIAL/EMOTIONAL DAILY LIVING SKILLS
        Self-concept/self-identity
            Knowing one's performance strengths and limitations
            Sensing one's competence, achievement, self-esteem, and self-respect
            Integrating new experiences with established self-concept/self-identity
        Situational coping
            Setting goals, selecting, harmonizing, and managing activities of daily living to promote optimal performance
            Perceiving changes and need for changes in self and environment
            Directing and redirecting energy to overcome problems
        Work
            Homemaking and home management tasks, such as meal planning, meal preparation, and clean-up
    COGNITIVE COMPONENTS
        Cognitive integration
            Generalization: generalize the skill and performance by applying specific concepts to a variety of related situations
            Problem solving the skill and performance by identifying and organizing solutions to difficulties organizing a plan

Form 3-6.
ACTIVITY ANALYSIS FORM

Student: _Example_ _____ Date: _____

Course: _____

Part I - Activity Summary
Directions: Respond to the following in list format.

1. Name of activity
   Sewing a button on a shirt

2. Brief description of activity
   The student will use a needle and thread to sew a button on the front of a shirt.

3. Tools/equipment (nonexpendable), cost and source
   Needle (package) — $1, scissors — $3, spool of thread — $.79, thimble — $1, pin (box) — $1.50, seam ripper — $2. Total cost of $9.29. sewing stores (JoAnn Fabrics, Cloth World,etc)

4. Materials/supplies (expendable), cost and source
   necessary materials include a button—$2.50, and thread (piece off the spool)—minimal cost. Total of $2.50. same as number 3

5. Space/environmental requirements
   The activity requires sitting in a chair, listening to the radio at a moderate sound level.

6. Sequence of major steps: time required for each step
   a. Unwrap thread from spool slowly: 10 sec.
   b. Cut thread carefully with scissors: 2 sec.
   c. Thread needle meticulously by placing end of thread through eye of needle: 3 min.
   d. Knot thread on end tightly: 20 sec.
   e. Position button precisely in correct spot on shirt: 30 sec.
   f. Place needle through hole in button from underside carefully: 35 sec.
   g. Continue over-under process arduously: 3-5 min.
   h. Tie end knot securely: 20 sec.
   i. Cut excess thread intently with scissors: 5 sec.

7. Precautions (review "Sequence of major steps")
   The student should wear a thimble and be careful with needle and scissors.

8. Contraindications (review participant's status)
   None

9. Special considerations (age appropriateness, educational requirements, cultural relevance, sexual identification, other)
   None

10. Acceptable criteria for completed project
    Button must be sewn on in appropriate place so that hole matches up and can be buttoned, and so that the button is secure enough that it will stay on.

Form 3-6. (continued)

Part II - Occupational Performance Components
Directions: Indicate the skill components necessary to complete the task (as it is normally done). State your reasoning to the right of each item. Write "N/A" if not applicable.

A. Sensorimotor Components
  1. Neuromuscular
     a. Reflex integration
        ATNR reflex and other primitive reflexes must be integrated to bring hands to midline and back out, in order to accomplish task of sewing.
     b. Range of motion
        (1) active
            Need complete control of muscle contractions and movement in order to sew
        (2) passive
            N/A
        (3) active assistive
            N/A
     c. Gross and fine coordination
        (1) muscle control
            Have to be able to control muscle movements to sew
        (2) coordination
            N/A
        (3) dexterity
            Need fine muscle control in order to thread needle and to manipulate needle to sew
     d. Strength and endurance
        (1) building strength, cardiopulmonary reserve
            N/A
        (2) increasing length of work period
            N/A
        (3) decreasing fatigue/strain
            N/A
  2. Sensory integration
     a. Sensory awareness
        (1) tactile awareness
            Ability to feel objects involved in sewing a button on the shirt
        (2) stereognosis
            Ability to identify needle in hand while under shirt
        (3) kinesthesia
            Needed to know where needle is being guided
        (4) proprioceptive awareness
            Need to know position of body in space in order to sew
        (5) ocular control
            Ability to focus on the sewing task
        (6) vestibular awareness
            Needed to maintain sitting position, balance, and head control
        (7) auditory awareness
            N/A
        (8) gustatory awareness
            N/A
        (9) olfactory awareness
            N/A

Form 3-6. (continued)

b. Visual-spatial awareness
  (1) figure-ground
  Needed in order to distinguish the shirt (background) from the button (foreground)
  (2) form constancy
  N/A
  (3) position in space
  Needed to know where body is in relation to sewing task
c. Body integration
  (1) body schema
  Needed to know where hand is in relation to the body while sewing
  (2) postural balance
  Needed to maintain balance and sitting position
  (3) bilateral motor coordination
  Needed to secure button with one hand and do the sewing motion in the other
  (4) right-left discrimination
  N/A
  (5) visual-motor integration
  Need hand-eye coordination to complete sewing task
  (6) crossing the midline
  Needed in order to bring needle through button
  (7) praxis
  Motor planning needed to carry out sewing task

B. Cognitive Components
  1. Orientation
  N/A
  2. Conceptualization/comprehension
    a. Concentration
    Need to mentally focus on task
    b. Attention span
    Needed to maintain concentration to complete sewing task
    c. Memory
    N/A
  3. Cognitive integration
    a. Generalization
    This could be generalized to other experiences of sewing a button on other garments
    b. Problem solving
      (1) defining or evaluating the problem
      Identify the necessity of a button on a shirt
      (2) organizing a plan
      Formulate steps needed to sew button on shirt
      (3) making decisions/judgment
      Decide on the color of the button and thread needed, and know when to stop sewing on button
      (4) implementing a plan
      Carrying out the organized steps to complete the sewing task
      (5) evaluating decision/judgment
      Evaluating how well the finished product looks

Form 3-6. (continued)

C. Psychosocial Components
  1. Self-management
    a. Self-expression
      (1) experiencing/recognizing a range of emotions
        N/A
      (2) having an adequate vocabulary
        N/A
      (3) writing and speaking skills
        N/A
      (4) use of nonverbal signs and symbols
        N/A
    b. Self-control
      (1) observing own and others' behavior
        Set mind to the task and use the appropriate behavior for sewing
      (2) recognizes need for change
        N/A
      (3) imitates new behavior
        N/A
      (4) directing energies into stress-reducing behaviors
        This should be a goal in any activity

  2. Dyadic interaction
    a. Understanding norms of communication and interaction
      N/A
    b. Setting limits on self and others
      N/A
    c. Compromising and negotiating
      N/A
    d. Handling stress
      N/A
    e. Cooperating and competing
      N/A
    f. Responsibly relying on self and others
      N/A

  3. Group interaction
    a. Performing social/emotional roles and tasks
      N/A
    b. Understanding simple group process
      N/A
    c. Participating in a mutually beneficial group
      N/A

Form 3-6. (continued)

D. Task Requirements
1. Work patterns
   a. Light
   It does not take much physical exertion to carry out sewing task

   b. Moderate
   N/A

   c. Heavy
   N/A

2. Method
   a. Structured
   N/A

   b. Methodical
   There is a method/way of sewing on a button correctly

   c. Repetitive
   There is repetition involved in going in and out of the holes in the button

   d. Expressive
   N/A

   e. Creative
   N/A

   f. Orderly
   The finished project should look neat (to wear)

   g. Physical contact
   N/A

   h. Projective
   The neatness and the way the button is sewn on could project the feelings of the individual (frustration, knots, messiness)

Form 3-6. (continued)

Part III - Occupational Performance
Directions: Indicate possible treatment goals that this activity might address in one or more of the areas of occupational performance. State your reasoning as in Part I. Write "N/A" if not applicable.

A. Independent Living/Daily Living Skills
   1. Physical daily living skills
      a. Grooming and hygiene
        N/A
      b. Feeding/eating
        N/A
      c. Dressing
        N/A
      d. Functional mobility
        N/A
      e. Functional communication
        N/A
      f. Object manipulation
        Manipulating needle, thread, and button involves fine motor coordination

   2. Psychological/emotional daily living skills
      a. Self-concept/self-identity
        N/A
      b. Situational coping
        N/A
      c. Community involvement
        N/A

   3. Work
      a. Homemaking
        Sewing a button on a shirt is a homemaking task
      b. Child care/parenting
        N/A
      c. Employment preparation
        N/A

   4. Play/leisure
      a. Recognizing one's needs
        N/A
      b. Identifying characteristics of play
        N/A
      c. Selecting play activities
        N/A
      d. Adaptation of activities
        N/A
      e. Utilizing community resources
        N/A

Form 3-6. (continued)

Part IV - Occupational Performance Modifications

Directions: Indicate ways this activity might be modified to increase independent function. State your reasoning. Write "N/A" if not applicable.

Note: This activity should be done with the non-dominant hand only.

A. Therapeutic Adaptations
    1. Orthotics
        a. Static or dynamic positioning
          N/A
        b. Relieve pain
          N/A
        c. Maintain joint alignment
          N/A
        d. Protect joint integrity
          N/A
        e. Improve function
          N/A
        f. Decrease deformity
          N/A
    2. Prosthetics
      N/A
    3. Assistive/adaptive equipment
        a. Architectural modification
          N/A
        b. Environmental modification
          N/A
        c. Assistive equipment
          Use a table that is at an appropriate level (adjustable table). While threading needle, put a piece of nonslip material on the bottom of styrofoam, then stick the needle in the styrofoam to stabilize the needle. This allows the nondominant hand to thread the needle. Use a magnifying glass to see eye of needle better. Use an embroidery loop to hold the material taut in the area being sewn. C-clamp the loop to the edge of a table for security.
        d. Wheelchair modification
          N/A

B. Prevention
    1. Energy conservation
        a. Energy-saving procedures
          Keeping all sewing materials in an organized sewing box. This prevents numerous trips to gather material.
        b. Activity restriction
          N/A
        c. Work simplification
          Refer to energy-saving procedures
        d. Time management
          Refer to energy-saving procedures
        e. Environmental organization
          Refer to energy-saving procedures

Form 3-6. (continued)

2. Joint protection/body mechanics
   a. Proper body mechanics
      N/A
   b. Avoiding static/deforming postures
      N/A
   c. Avoiding excessive weight bearing
      N/A
   d. Positioning
      Position chair within comfortable range of the sewing project.
   e. Coordination of daily living activities
      N/A

Implications for Treatment

Directions: Explain how and for whom this activity could be beneficial. Indicate physical and/or psychosocial dysfunction.

Physical: Use for people with upper extremity dysfunction; stroke—increase gross motor and fine motor coordination; hand injury—increase fine motor coordination; visually-impaired—increase independence.

Psychosocial: Use with psychiatric patients—directing concentration; use with depressed patients—engaging in purposeful activity to increase self-esteem.

Grading the Activity

Directions: Describe the ways you might grade this activity in terms of:

1. Duration/endurance
   Start with a base time and gradually increase the time spent on the sewing procedure
2. Range of motion
   Use different chair positions and table heights in relation to the project; use different thread lengths to increase range of motion of the shoulder
3. Resistance
   Use thicker needle; use wrist weights; use thicker thread
4. Complexity
   Use a smaller button or needle; use same color needle, thread, and material (figure-ground)
5. Independence
   Organize and carry out the procedure independently

Form 3-6a.
PATIENT-ACTIVITY CORRELATION FORM

Student: *Example (based on Profile 6 — Mike Marshall)*

Course: _____ Date: _____

1. Patient Profile
   Mike is a 19-year-old male with a diagnosis of moderate mental retardation. The client has been referred to occupational therapy for work preparation skills and self-care skills. He has progressed enough to be able to move from his parents' home to a group home. There, he will be responsible for all his self care. This includes arriving at his job site in clean, neat, and appropriate clothing.

2. Therapeutic Goals
   a. Long-term
      Job readiness skills with self-care preparation

   b. Short-term
      Sewing a button on a shirt

3. Goal-Directed Activity Description
   The client will use a needle and thread to sew a button on a shirt.

4. Activity Preparation Requirements
   a. Task
      N/A

   b. Personnel
      The primary therapist

   c. Preparation time
      It will take approximately 5 min. to gather the materials required to sew a button on a shirt (given the materials are in the occupational therapy department available for use).

   d. Place/space
      The equipment room in the occupational therapy department

   e. Materials
      N/A

   f. Equipment
      N/A

   g. Safety precautions (personnel)
      N/A

Form 3-6a. (continued)

5. Activity Implementation Requirements
    a. Personnel
       N/A
    b. Setting/location
       N/A
    c. Area/space
       To be done sitting comfortably in a chair beside a table in the occupational therapy department
    d. Environment
       To be done in an area of the occupational therapy department where distractions are minimal.
    e. Materials
       N/A
    f. Equipment/adaptations
       A needle, scissors, spool of thread, pin box, seam ripper, and button will be needed.
    g. Time frame
       N/A

    e. Safety precautions(patient)
       Safety guidelines should be provided to the client regarding use of the needle and scissors; check to make sure that the equipment needed is in the department ahead of time; and the client should be observed closely.

6. Activity Sequence (Action steps: ten or less)
    a. *The therapist presents a sewing box to the client along with a list of items needed for the task (can be words or pictures, depending on the cognitive level of the client).*
    b. *The client chooses the appropriate materials to carry out the task.*
    c. *The client unwraps and cuts the appropriate amount of thread to complete the task.*
    d. *The client threads the needle and knots the end of the thread in preparation for the sewing task.*
    e. *The client positions the button on the shirt in the appropriate place.*
    f. *The client places the needle through the button from the underside, and continues the over-under process 6-8 times. (This requires counting.)*
    g. *The client ties the end knot on the underneath side and cuts off excess thread with scissors.*
    h. *The finished product increases independence and self-esteem in the client.*

7. Therapeutic Application
   INDEPENDENT DAILY LIVING SKILLS
     Physical daily living skills
       Object manipulation: needed to use the needle
     Work
       Employment preparation: self care skills for job preparation
   SENSORIMOTOR
     Neuromuscular
       Gross and fine coordination needed for manipulation of the needle
   COGNITIVE (OCCUPATIONAL PERFORMANCE COMPONENTS)
     Conceptualization/comprehension
       Concentration needed to focus on the task
       Attention span needed to complete the task
       Memory needed to remember what needs to be done, and what has already been done

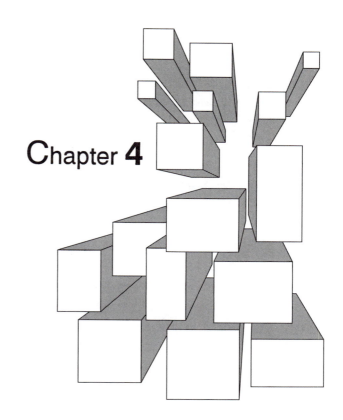

Chapter 4

INTEGRATING THE PROCESS

Learning Approach

Organizing the teaching/learning experience can be a challenge for both the instructor and the student. The following suggested approach is based on several years of working with the material. Both students and instructors agree that the material should be considered in small sections in order to lay a good groundwork for more extensive analysis and clinical application as the student progresses through the educational program.

1. Film: *Occupational Therapy: The Human Resource*. The American Occupational Therapy Association (AOTA).

   Comment: An overview of occupational therapy treatment at a modern, metropolitan medical center. The film serves as a point of reference for later discussion of the Occupational Performance Chart.

2. Definition: The definition of occupational therapy is used from Uniform Terminology For Reporting Occupational Therapy Services (see Appendix C) and the dictionary definition.

   Comment: A review and comparison of these two sources is helpful in establishing a knowledge base.

3. *Purposeful Activity: A Position Paper.* AOTA (see Appendix A)
Comment: Used as a reading assignment and a basis for lecture/discussion, this paper ensures that the student knows and understands the basis of purposeful activity in occupational therapy.

4. Activity Awareness Form
Comment: This may be completed during class using an activity performed by the student earlier in the day. Because this exercise attempts to capture the subconscious response to activity, no preparation or correlation with the concept of purposeful activity should be given immediately preceding its use.

5. Action Identification Form
Comment: The part labeled "Observation of Self" may be done in class using either the suggested activities listed in this section or one assigned by the instructor. The activity selected should be one that can be repeated by another person outside of class so the student can begin using observation and recording skills. Practice in using the Do-What-How format prior to the exercise is helpful. A discussion of the comparison of the way two people complete the same task should follow.

6. Uniform Terminology for Reporting Occupational Therapy Services (UTS) and UTS Revised (see Appendices C & D)
Comment: The student should be introduced to the origin and purpose of these documents as well as their checklists, headings, and definitions. Beginning with a simple activity, such as "walking on a sunny day," the student should work through the Occupational Performance Chart, noting the appropriate occupational performance area and selecting the corresponding performance components. The student may look at possible modifications of the activity as progress is made toward independent function. Students become eager to think about patient diagnoses at this point, but it is important to consider and be aware of normal, i.e., their own, performance of an activity.

7. Activity Analysis (AA) Form, Part I
Comment: In completing this section, several things need to be carefully considered. First, students should make responses as if they are doing the activity instead of a given patient. Second, the activity description sets the foundation for the rest of the analysis and must be stated in a focused and concrete manner. Only those skills that are required to complete the activity will be recorded in response to the position paper (see Appendix A). Third, the student needs to realistically consider the time needed to complete the treatment session. While the required steps of simple activities may be easily completed, the making of splints or leadership of a group is more demanding in terms of scheduling, preparation, and cost containment.

8. AA Form, Part II
Comment: Students should complete this section as if performing the activity themselves, i.e., as it is normally performed.

9. AA Form, Part III
Comment: The student considers how this activity may be applied to the three major performance areas (as done earlier in the exercise using the Occupational Performance Chart).

10. AA Form, Part IV
Comment: The student considers modifications of the activity, the way the activity might be used as a treatment modality, and how it may be graded to increase function or meet patient needs. This section may be considered in light of a personal disability such as using the nondominant hand to complete an activity.

11. Patient-Activity Correlation (PAC) Form Patient Profile

    Comment: The student is introduced to patient problems requiring occupational therapy intervention and considers the impact of the referral on treatment.

12. PAC Form, Long- and Short-term Goals

    Comment: The student focuses on the outcome of occupational therapy treatment using the profile and referral information provided above. In an initial exposure to this form, the student may be asked to formulate only one long- and one short-term goal. When the instructor is satisfied that the student can articulate the interdependence between the referral and goals, more goals can be required under both long- and short-term sections.

13. PAC Form, Activity Description

    Comment: An exact description of the activity to be used in treatment is important. What the therapist will do prior to the treatment session (Preparation), what the therapist will need to carry out the treatment session (Implementation), of what safety factors to be aware, and what symptoms to observe in a given patient (Precautions) must be identified.

14. PAC Form, Activity Sequence

    Comment: The student looks at the steps of performing the activity as they reflect and fulfill the requirements of the patient's referral needs and goals. The sequence of activity steps takes a therapeutic nature as the purpose of using the activity becomes apparent. This is an important transition for the beginning student to make in understanding the nature of activity as used in occupational therapy.

15. PAC Form, Therapeutic Application

    Comment: The student uses the vocabulary of UTS to describe the use of the activity for therapeutic intervention.

16. Film: *The Richness of Activity*. AOTA. Susan Fine, OTR, demonstrates theoretical concepts, activity history, activity analysis, and activity process in mental health using case histories as examples.

    Comment: This is a good tool for summarizing the need for and use of activity analysis. A showing of the film early in the coursework, followed by a later viewing, reveals the depth of knowledge and comprehension the student has achieved in understanding purposeful activity.

Final Comments: The activity analysis and patient-activity correlation can be effectively incorporated into media, daily life skills and group courses. They become second nature to the student the more they are used and build skills in treatment planning and documentation.

Thought Starters

Students can begin to think about occupational therapy and the roles activities play in making their own lives meaningful by answering one or more of the following.

1. Throughout life, we engage in activities. Recall an activity learned early in your life and reflect upon the significance that activity had when you:
   a. First attempted it
   b. Mastered it
   c. Forgot how or changed the way you did it

2. In examining the activities that take up your time now, place them in one of Gail Fidler's categories:
   a. Testing a skill
   b. Clarifying a relationship
   c. Creating an end product
3. "A reduction in activity generates pathology" (Fidler). Remember a time when you were physically ill and recall activities that you were unable to perform.
4. In your own words describe the difference between "Doing" and "Not doing anything." What is your response and the meaning of your answer to the query: "Are you doing anything tonight?"
5. Your decision "to live" and go on living is influenced by your perception that there are worthwhile activities that you specifically want to perform. Describe some of these activities at this time. If you physically, cognitively, or socially were unable to perform one of these activities, what would your response be?
6. Describe experiences that you have had with arts, crafts and hobbies since childhood. Identify which you liked most and which could be taught to other students. Repeat the process thinking of groups in which you have been involved.
7. To demonstrate a good comprehension of what occupational therapy is, describe "occupational therapy" to the following people (use vocabulary and content suitable to the anticipated interaction).
   a. An interested relative older than yourself.
   b. A potential patient younger than yourself.
   c. Another health professional of your own age.

Discussion Pointers

The following statements may be used to stimulate small group discussions about Activity Analysis and its uses. A pre- and post-test may be formed by modifying the statements and placing the phrases in multiple choice format.
1. In defining occupational therapy (OT), basic concepts are
   - OT is not directed at teaching specific job skills to individual workers
   - OT assists in the recovery of occupational skills
   - OT does not provide an employment service for the unemployed
   - OT deals with the mind and psychiatric problems
2. Occupational therapists use "purposeful activity" as a tool to treat individuals because
   - there is a relationship between health and activity
   - such activities help individuals become competent in work, self-care and play
   - the patient/client can become involved with the task rather than focusing on how or if he is able to perform it
   - the relationship of an activity to a purpose is made by using the professional judgment of the therapist
3. Characteristics of activities used in occupational therapy include their ability to
   - have significance to the patient/client
   - be directed or structured to fit the purpose desired
   - vary in complexity and the amount of time and strength required
   - be determined through the OT's professional judgment as meaningful and effective in reaching therapeutic goals

4. Assumptions about the use of activity in OT include
   - activity provides a way of exploring the world and developing self-awareness
   - normal growth and development involve activity
   - several systems of functioning including cognitive, motor, and psychosocial areas which are integrated in doing activities
   - activity provides a sense of well-being for the individual, especially when used in a therapeutic manner

5. An activity selected for use in OT treatment may be geared to
   - improve or maintain function of the person
   - lengthen the life span of an individual
   - prevent malfunction of the body part
   - provide financial compensation for the patient/client

6. The occupational therapist is trained in the analysis of activities because activity analysis
   - specifies therapeutic benefits of an activity and contributes information to justify its use
   - provides the therapist with a knowledge base for instructing patients how to do an activity
   - helps the therapist determine for whom the activity would be therapeutic
   - can be used to justify and document patient treatment

7. When deciding on an activity to be used in treatment, the therapist should be able to
   - determine the location for the activity
   - describe a therapeutic rationale for using the activity with a patient
   - know and do the activity well enough to instruct others
   - select the activity that intervenes in the most beneficial way for the patient

8. When choosing an activity for the patient, the therapist
   - may make an independent decision, but attempts to involve the patient in the decision-making process
   - considers the patient's interests of primary importance to therapeutic goals
   - seeks out activities suitable to the patient's age, sex and socioeconomic level
   - correlates the activity to specific treatment outcomes

9. An OT can benefit a patient/client by
   - preventing the loss of skills in a person or developing skills not present
   - using adapted methods of performing skills
   - maintaining skills at an established level of performance
   - enhancing the quality of life for the patient/client

10. An activity used in OT is determined through the therapist's professional judgment based on knowledge. This implies that
    - schooling in OT is required to become qualified to select activities appropriately
    - the knowledge learned in OT equips the therapist with skills to correlate meaningful activities with patient needs
    - the ability to judge and assess the therapeutic value of activities is part of the uniqueness of the OT profession
    - understanding the value of activity, when choosing activities which are to be used therapeutically, is of major importance

11. When choosing an activity for a patient with a physical disability, the activity should
    - provide for the alternate contraction and relaxation of muscles
    - permit repeated use of the desired movement

- allow a gradation in the amount of resistance, coordination and change in joint range needed
- be selected to reflect normal activity

12. An activity in OT that is said to be goal directed means the activity is
    - not "busy work" to keep the patient occupied
    - specific to the patient or his needs
    - purposeful and of value to the patient
    - not a game where the highest number of points scored wins

13. An activity used in OT treatment must have significance to the client at some level. This means the activity
    - has some relationship to the client's roles in life
    - is of some use to the client even though not immediately experienced
    - has real importance to the client and is of personal value
    - may make it possible for the client to reach a goal

14. An activity that reflects patient involvement in life task situations involves
    - developing competencies in the skills a patient must have to resume life roles
    - using, redeveloping or acquiring skills needed to return to society
    - work, play or daily life skills
    - some area of independent function

15. A patient-activity correlation is used to
    - look at the major contributions of an activity
    - help match patient needs with an activity's potential for use in treatment
    - incorporate Uniform Terminology to report therapy outcomes
    - clarify long- and short-term goals related to the use of a specific activity

16. When selecting an activity to use in the treatment of a patient, the occupational therapist should consider
    - the amount of time involved in doing the activity
    - the type of learning required to do the activity
    - the property of the materials used in the activity
    - the number of steps in the activity

17. An activity that is adaptable and gradable means the activity may be
    - changed to fit the client's needs
    - increased or decreased in the complexity of steps involved
    - flexible in its requirements of time, strength or range of motion
    - modified to suit age, culture or social preferences

18. An activity used in OT treatment that relates to the client's interests considers
    - involving the client in the choice of the activity
    - meeting the client's goals
    - the client's commitment to doing the activity
    - eliciting the client's interest

19. The Uniform Terminology System (UTS) is an important document for use in reporting occupational therapy services because
    - it describes treatment in terms of results instead of in terms of the modalities used
    - it reflects the terms and definitions used in Medicare and Medicaid guidelines
    - it is universally accepted by physicians and insurance companies to describe OT services
    - it portrays the uniqueness of the OT profession when compared with other professional services

Review Questions

These questions highlight and provide an overview of the learning designed to take place when using this textbook. The nature of the questions implies an essay-type response, but may be used effectively in group study sessions.

1. What is an Activity Analysis (AA) and why is it important?
2. What are some specific reasons for performing an AA?
3. How does the Uniform Terminology System (UTS) correlate with the use of AA?
4. What kinds of information can AA provide to teach activities to patients experiencing visual problems? Hearing problems? Loss of sensation? Use of one hand? Limited mobility?
5. How can AA help a therapist determine measurable criteria to evaluate a patient's progress?
6. How can AA be used in the inventory process of an OT clinic? In planning new OT departments? In determining storage and space requirements? In upgrading facilities?
7. Why does the profession have UTS?
8. What are the major categories of UTS and how do they compare to OT Performance Areas?
9. What are the main components OTs look at in each performance area?
10. What advantages does the UTS provide the therapist charting a patient's progress?
11. What factors should the therapist consider in selecting an activity to meet the patient's progress?
12. What are the characteristics of an activity used in OT treatment?
13. What is a Patient-Activity Correlation and how does it differ from an Activity Analysis?
14. What does the phrase "health through activity" mean to an OT?

Learning Experiences

For Further Exploration

To increase awareness of activity as a life organizer and the occupational nature of human beings, one or more of the following activities are suggested.

1. Perform an activity configuration and make observations based on the data collected.
2. Analyze a 5-year timeline on one's life in whatever way is most meaningful and present this in written form.
3. Compose an artistic representation of a human occupation through art, music, creative writing, drama, etc.
4. Explore an occupation by reading about it and then observing someone engaged in it. Record some of the activities specific to this job and choose one to learn as a new skill.
5. Plan and implement a group social function of your choice and write a brief description of the following:
   a. Plans made for the event.
   b. Tasks completed to make the event happen.
   c. The actual event as it took place (describe what really happened).

d. Critique of the process. Mention participant's reactions and your own feelings concerning the activities that occurred.

Events may take a variety of forms (birthday party, group hike, family visit, religious function, study session, etc.).

Occupational Therapy Performance Areas

These two exercises may be used in lab or media classes as group activities to promote general understanding of skills used in completing daily life tasks and the performance components involved.

General Task Breakdown

Choose an occupational therapy performance-related task and describe it in one sentence. For example: under work activities, count out ten envelopes and bind them with a rubber band or file address cards in alphabetical order by last name. Break down the task to answer the following questions.

1. What is the best method of doing this task? Consider the layout of materials and supplies, placement of the finished task, the number of people needed to perform the task cost effectively, and the number of steps needed to complete the task efficiently.

2. How could you instruct a patient to perform this task? Consider the Do-What-How format, verbal and nonverbal cues that could be provided, prompts and wording of instructions (written and/or verbal).

3. What skills and knowledge are prerequisites to perform this task? To learn this task? How could the task be modified to accommodate age and/or gender preferences?

Specific Task Breakdown

Choose one task in a specific occupational performance area and describe it in one sentence. For example: a parent preparing a lunch meal for children or an employee punching a timecard.

List performance components needed to do the task as described in UTS and the reason that component is needed. For example in managing a home, one of the tasks to be performed is taking out the garbage. Performance components needed to complete the task include

- gross and fine motor skills to lift out the garbage bag and apply a wire twist tie around the bag opening
- praxis to motor plan movements and keep the garbage from spilling from the bag
- visual ground discrimination to discern the edge of the bag to fasten the tie, etc.

Compare your thoughts with another examining the same task.

Patient-Activity Correlation Experiential

Objectives

1. Given a specific case study, the student should be able to:
   a. Identify the expected functional loss of the patient in relation to sensorimotor, cognitive, and psychosocial performance.
   b. Determine the implications for ability to perform a particular activity based on a diagnostic group.
   c. Role-play a teaching session with a "patient" having that dysfunction.

    d. Complete a patient-activity correlation based on the case—study and role-play situation.

Method for Accomplishing Objectives

1. Read Willard & Spackman's *Occupational Therapy-Base in Activity.* (7th edition) pp. 93-101.
2. Review class notes.
3. Investigate the specific diagnosis described in the case study for symptoms, patient needs, and functional expectations.
4. Select an activity (discussed in class) appropriate for this particular patient/client.
5. Arrange with another student to role-play as the patient for your teaching session.
6. Structure a teaching session indicating objectives, teaching methods, steps of instruction and expected outcomes (can be given orally prior to teaching session).
7. Independently procure tools and materials necessary to perform an activity, produce aids to learning, and arrange setting for a teaching role-play session.
8. Role play a teaching session with a "patient" having that dysfunction.
9. Complete and submit to the instructor a patient-activity correlation based on the case study and role-play situation.
10. Attach to the patient-activity correlation your self-evaluation of the teaching session, based on peer evaluations and your own assessment.

Helpful Suggestions

1. Practice the activity prior to teaching session.
2. Do a dress rehearsal; in other words, organize your role-play session with your "patient" so as to eliminate unexpected problems.
3. Allow time for preparation, set-up, and clean-up.
4. Prior to the teaching session, set the stage for the audience with a brief description of the activity and patient diagnosis. See method #6.
5. Provide motivational cues to the "patient."

Forty Diagnostic Categories for Patient-Activity Correlation

1. Cerebral vascular accident, (R) hemiplegia with expressive aphasia, 52-year-old male civil engineer, married, with two children in their 20s.
2. Advanced Parkinson's Disease, 78-year-old female living in a long-term care facility, widow with one daughter, ambulates with difficulty and tires easily.
3. Senile dementia, 80-year-old female living in a nursing home where her husband visits daily.
4. Diabetes, 68-year-old female widow with four grown children; enjoys handiwork.
5. Hip fracture (R), 75-year-old male in hospital for eight weeks with emphasis on Daily Living Skills before being discharged to home. Married.
6. Mental retardation, 35-year-old female, with short attention span; hyperactive, annoying to other patients.
7. Manic-depressive, 30-year-old female homemaker and mother of two preschool children; few vocational skills.
8. Moderate mentally retarded adolescent prescribed prevocational exploration.
9. Mild Parkinson's, 60-year-old male widower, retired railroad engineer.
10. Multiple sclerosis, 40-year-old female with incoordination of upper extremities and low fatigue level.

11. Situational adjustment reaction, 35-year-old male, a carpenter by trade; low self-esteem.
12. Below-knee amputation (resulting from industrial accident), 25-year-old male, single, wants to return to previous job.
13. Myocardial infarction, 50-year-old male, family includes wife and three school-age children; businessman with few leisure interests.
14. Cerebral vascular accident, (L) hemiparesis, 65-year-old female with short attention span and perceptual impairment.
15. Depression, 25-year-old female, secretary, single.
16. Learning disability, 18-year-old male with poor vocational skills but good family support.
17. Paraplegia (resulting from diving accident), 17-year-old male, college-bound with interest in computers.
18. Cerebral palsy, mixed athetosis and spasticity, wheelchair-bound 16-year-old female with average intelligence.
19. Closed-head injury, 25-year-old male with disorientation and perceptual impairment, family includes wife and infant, worked as newspaper artist.
20. Head injury, 45-year-old male, with poor grasp and weak pronation, industrial accident, wants to return to job.
21. Cancer, terminal, 55-year-old female with husband and two grown children, former bank teller.
22. Rheumatoid arthritis with involvement of wrists and hands, 56-year-old female, widow and schoolteacher.
23. Second degree burns, 26-year-old male, burned on face, chest, and forearms, now on rehab unit, mail carrier.
24. Depression, 18-year-old female, with suicidal tendencies, poor social environment, needs prevocational evaluation.
25. Guillian-Barre Syndrome, 31-year-old male electrical engineer, married with no children, limited upper extremity strength and endurance.
26. Multiple sclerosis, 29-year-old male carpenter, married with 2$\frac{1}{2}$-year-old daughter, fair upper extremity/muscle strength but wheelchair-bound.
27. Paraplegia, 34-year-old male truck driver.
28. Chronic schizophrenia, 35-year-old female with poor academic and social skills and low frustration tolerance.
29. Anorexia nervosa, 15-year-old female, admitted to general hospital in weakened condition, withdrawn, good academic skills.
30. Thumb injury (R), 40-year-old male involved in industrial accident, hopes to return to previous employment.
31. Carpal tunnel syndrome, 35-year-old female homemaker with two school-age children.
32. Visual impairment, 15-year-old female with good academic skills, admitted to hospital for eye surgery.
33. Cerebral vascular accident with (R) hemiparesis, 70-year-old female living alone, hopes to return to her apartment.
34. Diabetes, 15-year-old female, admitted to hospital for education for diabetes.
35. Cancer, arrested, 35-year-old female, married secretary, no children.
36. Brachial plexus injury, 60-year-old male retired salesman.
37. Rheumatoid arthritis, 42-year-old female homemaker with two school-age children.
38. Emphysema, 57-year-old businessman, married, preparing for retirement.

39. Brain tumor, causing pain and fatigue, 32-year-old female computer operator, single.
40. Anxiety reaction, 20-year-old male college student studying architecture.

The Application of PAC to a Case Study

Form 4-1 ties the Patient-Activity Correlation (PAC) to a specific patient. It provides the opportunity to apply principles of Activity Analysis in a case study situation. The patient may be hypothetical or one the student has observed as part of a supervised fieldwork experience. Guest lecturers can be encouraged to follow this format when presenting clinical information.

The form for completing this assignment is found in Appendix D (Student Worksheets).

Form 4-1.
APPLICATION OF PATIENT-ACTIVITY CORRELATION TO A CASE STUDY

1. Patient Profile

    a. Personal data:
       (1) Age _____ Sex _____ Marital Status _____
       (2) Occupation: _____
       (3) Diagnosis: _____

    b. Medical history (etiology, prognosis, symptomatology, medical and ancillary treatment)

    c. Screening/evaluation procedures

2. Therapeutic Goals: Long- and Short-term

3. Treatment Modalities

4. Progress

5. Discharge Summary

6. Following the presentation the student will determine Uniform Terminology
    a. Occupational performance area(s)

    b. Occupational performance components

7. Roles
    a. OTR

    b. COTA

References

American Occupational Therapy Association. *OTA Faculty Guide,* Role of occupational therapy with the elderly. Module III: Treatment approaches. Teaching Resource 65:131.

Cynkin, S. (1979). Occupational therapy toward health through activities. *Activity Configuration Protocol, 125,* 131. (1971).

Fidler, G.S. & Fidler, J.W. (1978). Doing and becoming: Purposeful action and self-actualization. *American Journal of Occupational Therapy, 32*(5), 305-310.

Watanabe, S. (1971). Activity configuration. In: Willard, H.S., Spackman, C.S. (Eds.) *Occupational Therapy, 4th Edition* (pp. 88-89). Philadelphia, PA: J.B. Lippincott Co.

Appendix **A**

PURPOSEFUL ACTIVITY
A POSITION PAPER

Jim Hinojosa, MA, OTR
Joyce Sabari, MA, OTR
Mark S. Rosenfeld, MS, OTR
in collaboration with:
Diane Shapiro, MS, OTR

The American Occupational Therapy Association, Inc., submits this paper to clarify the use of the term "purposeful activities" with regard to occupational therapy. Occupational therapists are committed to the use of purposeful activities.[1] Purposeful activity is an important legitimate tool used by occupational therapists to evaluate, facilitate, restore, and maintain function.[2]

Individuals engage in purposeful activity as part of their daily life routine. Purposeful activity, in this natural context, can be defined as tasks or experiences in which the person actively participates. Engagement in purposeful activity requires and elicits coordination between one's physical, emotional, and cognitive systems. An individual who is involved in purposeful activity directs attention to the task itself, rather than to the internal processes required for achievement of the task.

Activities may yield immediate results or require sustained effort and multiple repetition. They may represent novel and singular responses or be part of complex long-standing patterns of behavior.[3] Purposeful activities, influenced by the individual's life roles, have unique meaning to each person.[4]

Occupational therapists treat individuals whose capacity to function effectively is impaired due to injury, illness, psychosocial stress, changing developmental and environmental demands, or lack of skill. This impairment can diminish an individuals's ability to produce, have positive self-image, or perform life-enriching activities, and can affect the ability to fulfill desired life roles.

Occupational therapy education in activity analysis and the behavioral and biological sciences provide the background necessary to use activities as therapeutic modalities for clients with a variety of physical, cognitive, emotional, and social disorders. Occupational therapists evaluate clients to determine an individual's activity goals, the capacity to plan and perform purposeful activities, and the ability to meet the functional demands of the environment.

Based on this evaluation, the occupational therapist designs activity experiences that offer the client opportunities for effective action. These activities are purposeful in that they assist and build upon the individual's abilities and lead to achievement of personal goals.

A purposeful activity, as used by the occupational therapist, leads to the fulfillment of simultaneous goals. One may be the client's goal to complete the overall task satisfactorily. The other may be identified by the occupational therapist as: to promote balance, increase muscle strength, increase attention span. The activity is in itself an end, as well as being a means to a larger end.[5]

Occupational therapists divide activities into component parts to determine which skills are necessary to complete the task. This information allows the occupational therapist to adapt, grade, and combine activities into therapeutic modalities.

Occupational therapists adapt activities in different ways to promote performance. Activities are adapted by modifying or changing the sequence of the activity, or both, such as the position of the client, the position of the material, the size, shape, weight, or texture of the material, the procedures, and the nature and degree of interpersonal contact. Adaptation involves the process of continually modifying an activity to meet the specific changing needs of the client.

In each individual situation, occupational therapists determine whether the activity will be adapted to compensate for a functional deficit, or to promote restoration. This decision is based on the extent of the client's disability, as well as their current level of performance. Purposeful activities cannot be routinely prescribed.

Occupational therapists may present a series of activities, or change the steps within the activity. Such grading provides skill development and therapeutic exercise to respond to the dynamic changes of the client.

Occupational therapists artfully modify routine activities within the client's daily life in order to promote psychological or physical development. At first, functional tasks may be introduced in a controlled environment. As treatment progresses, the occupational therapist gradually changes the environment until the client demonstrates the level of skills necessary to function in their real life environment.[6]

Occupational therapists use current rehabilitation procedures to enhance a client's skill development or task performance. Throughout the activity, occupational therapists modify their method of personal interaction to achieve the desired results of the activity.

In summary, occupational therapists enable individuals to engage in purposeful activities to achieve competence in work, self-care, and play/leisure. Activities provide direct and objective feedback about the client's performance, both to the occupational therapist and to the client. Successful performance of purposeful activities promotes feelings of competence and provides opportunities for individuals to achieve mastery of their environments.[7]

Purposeful activities involve the "doing processes which require the use of thought and energy and are directed toward an intended or desired end."[8]

References

1. *Philosophical Base of Occupational Therapy.* Adopted by Representative Assembly of The American Occupational Therapy Association in Denver, 1979.
2. Mosey, A.C. (1981). *Occupational Therapy-Configuration of a Profession.* Chapter 10, New York, Raven Press.
3. Cynkin, S. (1979). *Occupational Therapy: Toward Health Through Activities.* Boston: Little, Brown & Co.
4. Predretti, L.W. *The compatibility of current treatment methods in physical disabilities with the philosophical base of occupational therapy.* Presentation at The American Occupational Therapy Association Annual Conference in Philadelphia, May 1982.
5. King, L.J. (1978). Toward a science of adaptive responses. *American Journal of Occupational Therapy, 32,* 429-437.
6. Rogers, J.C. (1982). The spirit of independence: the evolution of a philosophy. *American Journal of Occupational Therapy, 36,* 709-715.
7. Fidler, G.S. (1981). From crafts to competence. *American Journal of Occupational Therapy, 35,* 567-573.
8. Mosey, A.C. Purposeful Activities. Unpublished paper.

Adopted April 1983 by the Representative Assembly, The American Occupational Therapy Association, Inc. Used by permission of The American Occupational Therapy Association.

Appendix B

UNIFORM TERMINOLOGY FOR REPORTING OCCUPATIONAL THERAPY SERVICES,
FIRST EDITION

*Commission on Practice, the American Occupational Therapy Association, Inc.
Adopted March 1979 by The Representative Assembly, AOTA
Used by permission of the American Occupational Therapy Association, Inc., Rockville, Maryland.

Introduction

August 1978, the American Occupational Therapy Association Executive Board charged the Commission on Practice to form a Task Force to 1) review the existing occupational therapy terminology and relative value reporting systems, and 2) develop a proposal for a national occupational therapy product output reporting system.

At the time Public Law 95–142 was passed, no national system for reporting productivity of hospital based occupational therapy services existed. The American Occupational Therapy Association Commission on Practice OT Uniform Reporting System Task Force was created in August 1978 to develop a proposal for a national system. Sylvia Harlock, OTR (Washington), member of the AOTA Commission on Practice, was appointed by the Commission Chair, John Farace, OTR, to chair the Task Force.

Members selected to serve on the Task Force were:

Mary Lou Hymen, OTR	California
Kathy McFarland, OTR	Washington
Kathy Saunders, OTR	Wisconsin
Louise Thibodaux, OTR	Alabama
Carole Hays, OTR	Division on Practice, AOTA National Office

Description of Occupational Therapy Service. Given the diversity of services provided by occupational therapy, the multiplicity of evaluation and treatment procedures which may often be used to achieve the same treatment outcomes, and the lack of a uniformly used description of occupational therapy service delivery, including definitions of terminology, the Task Force first developed the Description of Occupational Therapy Services. In selecting items and defining terms, the following criteria were taken into consideration:

1. Emphasis on description of treatment outcomes rather than treatment procedures.
2. Reflection of Medicare and Medicaid guidelines in terminology and category selection and definition.
3. Comprehensive description of occupational therapy services/product.
4. Reflection of the uniqueness of occupational therapy services/product in comparison with the services of other professions.
5. Coverage of recognized occupational therapy role in medical practice rather than all possible occupational therapy roles.

Occupational Therapy Function

Occupational Therapy is the application of purposeful, goal—oriented activity in the evaluation, problem identification, and/or treatment of persons whose function is impaired by physical illness or injury, emotional disorder, congenital or developmental disability, or the aging process, in order to achieve optimum functioning, to prevent disability, and to maintain health. Specific occupational therapy services include, but are not limited to the following:

education and training and evaluation of performance capacity in activities of daily living (ADL); the design, fabrication, and application of orthoses (splints); sensorimotor activities; guidance in selection and use of adaptive equipment; therapeutic use of activities and the *activity process* to develop/restore function performance; prevocational evaluation and training; consultation concerning the adaptation of physical environments for the handicapped; involvement in discharge planning and community re–entry; time/space/role management; and opportunity for self–expression and communication. These services are provided to individuals, groups, and to the community.

Occupational Therapy Services
Outline

I. Occupational Therapy Assessment
  A. Screening
  B. Patient–Related Consultation
  C. Evaluation
    1. Independent Living/Daily Living Skills and Performance
    2. Sensorimotor Skill and Performance Components
    3. Cognitive Skill and Performance Components
    4. Psychosocial Skill and Performance Components
    5. Therapeutic Adaptations
    6. Specialized Evaluation
  D. Reassessment

II. Occupational Therapy Treatment
  A. Independent Living/Daily Living Skills
    1. Physical Daily Living Skills
      a. Grooming and Hygiene
      b. Feeding/Eating
      c. Dressing
      d. Functional Mobility
      e. Functional Communication
      f. Object Manipulation
    2. Psychological/Emotional Daily Living Skills
      a. Self–concept/Self–identity
      b. Situational Coping
      c. Community Involvement
    3. Work
      a. Homemaking
      b. Child Care/Parenting
      c. Employment Preparation
    4. Play/Leisure
  B. Sensorimotor Components
    1. Neuromuscular
      a. Reflex Integration
      b. Range of Motion
      c. Gross and Fine Coordination
      d. Strength and Endurance
    2. Sensory Integration
      a. Sensory Awareness
      b. Visual–Spatial Awareness
      c. Body Integration
  C. Cognitive Components
    1. Orientation
    2. Conceptualization/Comprehension
      a. Concentration
      b. Attention Span
      c. Memory

        3. Cognitive Integration
          a. Generalization
          b. Problem Solving
      D. Psychosocial Components
        1. Self–Management
          a. Self–Expression
          b. Self–Control
        2. Dyadic Interaction
        3. Group Interaction
      E. Therapeutic Adaptation
        1. Orthotics
        2. Prosthetics
        3. Assistive/Adaptive Equipment
      F. Prevention
        1. Energy Conservation
        2. Joint Protection/Body Mechanics
        3. Positioning
        4. Coordination of Daily Living Skills

III. Patient/Client–Related Conferences
    A. Professional Conference
    B. Agency Conferences
    C. Patient/Client–Advocate Conferences

IV. Travel: Patient Treatment Related

The following items do not involve direct patient care.

V. Service Management
    A. Quality Review/Maintenance of Quality
        1. Development of Standards of Quality Treatment/Services
        2. Chart Audit
        3. Accrediting Reviews
        4. Occupational Therapy Care Review
        5. Inservice Education
    B. Departmental Maintenance
    C. Employee Meetings
    D. Program–Related Conferences
    E. Supervision

VI. Education
    A. Occupational Therapy Clinical Education: Occupational Therapy Students
    B. Occupational Therapy Clinical Education: Others
    C. Continuing Education

VII. Research

Occupational Therapy Services
Description

I. *OCCUPATIONAL THERAPY ASSESSMENT*

Occupational therapy assessment refers to the process of determining the need for, nature of, and estimated time of treatment, determining the needed coordination with other persons involved, and documenting these activities.

A. *Screening*

Screening refers to the review of potential patient's/client's case to determine the need for evaluation and treatment. It includes discussion with other professionals and/or patient advocate, and patient/client interview or administration of screening tool.

B. *Patient–Related Consultation*

Patient–related consultation refers to the sharing of relevant information with other professionals of patients/clients who are not currently referred to occupational therapy. This may include but is not limited to discussion, chart review, treatment recommendation, and documentation.

C. *Evaluation*

Evaluation refers to the process of obtaining and interpreting data necessary for treatment. This includes planning for and documenting the evaluation process and results. This data may be gathered through record review, specific observation, interview, and the administration of data collection procedures. Such procedures include but are not limited to the use of standardized tests, performance checklists, and activities and tasks designed to evaluate specific performance abilities. Categories of occupational therapy evaluation include independent living/daily living skills and performance and their components.

1. *Independent Living/Daily Living Skills and Performance (see II A).*
2. *Sensorimotor Skill and Performance Components (see II B).*
3. *Cognitive Skill and Performance Components (see II C).*
4. *Psychosocial Skill and Performance Components (see II D).*
5. *Therapeutic Adaptations (see II E).*
6. *Specialized Evaluations.*

Specialized evaluations refer to evaluations or tests requiring specialized training and/or advanced education to administer and interpret. Examples of specialized evaluations are employment preparation, evaluation (prevocational testing), sensory integration evaluation, prosthetic evaluation, driver's training evaluation.

D. *Reassessment*

Reassessment refers to the process of obtaining and interpreting data necessary for updating treatment plans and goals. This frequently involves administering only portions of the initial evaluation, documenting results, and/or revising treatment.

II. *OCCUPATIONAL THERAPY TREATMENT*

Occupational therapy treatment refers to the use of specific activities or methods to develop, improve, and/or restore the performance of necessary functions; compensate for dysfunction; and/or minimize debilitation; and the planning for and documenting of treatment performance. The necessary functions treated in occupational therapy are the following:

A. *Independent Living/Daily Living Skills*
1. *Physical Daily Living Skills*
   Physical daily living skills refer to the skill and performance of daily personal care, with or without adaptive equipment. It includes but is not limited to:
   a. *Grooming and Hygiene*
       Grooming and hygiene refer to the skill and performance of personal health needs, such as bathing, toileting, hair care, shaving, applying make-up.
   b. *Feeding/Eating*
       Feeding/eating refers to the skill and performance of sequentially feeding oneself, including sucking, chewing, swallowing, and using appropriate utensils.
   c. *Dressing*
       Dressing refers to the skill and performance of choosing appropriate clothing, dressing oneself in a sequential fashion, including fastening and adjusting clothing.
   d. *Functional Mobility*
       Functional mobility refers to the skill and performance in moving oneself from one position or place to another. It includes skills necessary for activities such as bed mobility, wheelchair mobility, transfers (bed, car, tub, toilet, chair), and functional ambulation, with or without adaptive aids. It also includes use of public and private travel systems, such as driving own automobile and using public transportation.
   e. *Functional Communication*
       Functional communication refers to the skill and performance in using equipment or systems to enhance or provide communication, such as writing equipment, typewriters, letterboards, telephone, braille writers, artificial vocalization systems and computers.
   f. *Object Manipulation*
       Object manipulation refers to the skill and performance in handling large and small common objects, such as calculators, keys, money, light switches, doorknobs, and packages.
2. *Psychological/Emotional Daily Living Skills*
   Psychological/emotional daily living skills refers to the skill and performance in developing one's self–concept/self–identity, coping with life situations, and participating in one's organizational and community environment. It includes but is not limited to:
   a. *Self–concept/Self–identity*
       Self–concept/self–identity refers to the cognitive image of one's functional self. This includes but is not limited to:
       (1) clearly perceiving one's needs, feelings, conflicts, values, beliefs, expectations, sexuality, and power.
       (2) realistically perceiving others' needs, feelings, conflicts, values, beliefs, expectations, sexuality, and power.
       (3) knowing one's performance strengths and limitations.
       (4) sensing one's competence, achievement, self–esteem, and self–respect.
       (5) integrating new experiences with established self–concept/self–identity.
       (6) having a sense of psychological safety and security.
       (7) perceiving one's goals and directions.

b. *Situational Coping*

Situational coping refers to skill and performance in handling stress and dealing with problems and changes in a manner that is functional for self and others. This includes but is not limited to:

(1) setting goals, selecting, harmonizing, and managing activities of daily living to promote optimal performance.

(2) testing goals and perceptions against reality.

(3) perceiving changes and need for changes in self and environment.

(4) directing and redirecting energy to overcome problems.

(5) initiating, implementing, and following through on decisions.

(6) assuming responsibility for self and consequences of actions.

(7) interacting with others, dyadic and group.

c. *Community Involvement*

Community involvement refers to skill and performance in interacting within one's social system. This includes but is not limited to:

(1) understanding social norms and their impact on society.

(2) planning, organizing, and executing daily life activities in relationship to society, including such activities as budgeting, time management, social role management, arranging for housing, nutritional planning, assessing and using community resources.

(3) recognizing and responding to needs to families, groups, and complex social units.

(4) understanding and responding to organizational/community role expectations as both recipient and contributor.

3. *Work*

Work refers to skill and performance in participating in socially purposeful and productive activities. These activities may take place in the home, employment setting, school, or community. They include but are not limited to:

a. *Homemaking*

Homemaking refers to skill and performance in homemaking and home management tasks, such as meal planning, meal preparation and clean–up, laundry, cleaning, minor household repairs, shopping, and use of household safety principles.

b. *Child Care/Parenting*

Child care/parenting refers to skill and performance in child care activities and management. This includes but is not limited to physical care of children, and use of age–appropriate activities, communication, and behavior to facilitate child development.

c. *Employment Preparation*

Employment preparation refers to skill and performance in precursory job activities (including prevocational activities). This includes but is not limited to:

(1) job acquisition skills and performance.

(2) organizational and team participatory skills and performance.

(3) work process skills and performance.

(4) work product quality.

4. *Play/Leisure*

Play/leisure refers to skill and performance in choosing, performing, and engaging in activities for amusement, relaxation, spontaneous enjoyment, and/or self-expression. This includes but is not limited to:

a. recognizing one's specific needs, interests, and adaptations necessary for performance.

b. identifying characteristics of activities and social situations that make them play for the individual.

c. identifying activities that contain those characteristics.

d. choosing play activities for participation, such as sports, games, hobbies, music, drama, and other activities.

e. testing out and adapting activities to enable participation.

f. identifying and using community resources.

B. *Sensorimotor Components*

Sensorimotor components refer to the skill and performance of patterns of sensory and motor behavior that are prerequisites to self-care, work, and play/leisure performance. The components in this section include neuromuscular and sensory integrative skills, including perceptual motor skills.

1. *Neuromuscular*

Neuromuscular refers to the skill and performance of motor aspects of behavior. This includes but is not limited to:

a. *Reflex Integration*

Reflex integration refers to skill and performance in enhancing and supporting functional neuromuscular development through eliciting and/or inhibiting stereotyped, patterned, and/or involuntary responses coordinated at subcortical and cortical levels.

b. *Range of Motion*

Range of motion refers to skill and performance in using maximum span of joint movement in activities with and without assistance to enhance functional performance. The standard levels of performance include:

(1) active range of motion: movement by patient, unassisted through a complete range of motion.

(2) passive range of motion: movement performed by someone other than patient or by a mechanical device, requiring no muscle contraction on the part of the patient.

(3) active-assistive range of motion: movement performed by the patient to the limit of his/her ability, and then completed with assistance.

c. *Gross and Fine Coordination*

Gross and fine coordination refers to skill and performance in muscle control, coordination, and dexterity while participating in activities.

(1) *muscle control*

muscle control refers to skill and performance in directing muscle movement.

(2) *coordination*

Coordination refers to skill and performance in gross motor activities using several muscle groups.

(3) *dexterity*

Dexterity refers to skill and performance in tasks using small muscle groups.

d. *Strength and Endurance*

Strength and endurance refers to skill and performance in using muscular force within time periods necessary for purposeful task performance.

lar force within time periods necessary for purposeful task performance. This involves but is not limited to progressively building strength and cardia and pulmonary reserve, increasing the length of work periods, and decreasing fatigue and strain.

2. *Sensory Integration*

Sensory integration refers to skill and performance in development and coordination of sensory input, motor output, and sensory feedback. This includes but is not limited to:

a. *Sensory Awareness*

Sensory awareness refers to skill and performance in perceiving and differentiating external and internal stimuli, such as:

(1) tactile awareness: the perception and interpretation of stimuli through skin contact.

(2) stereognosis: the identification of forms and nature of objects through the sense of touch.

(3) kinesthesia: the conscious perception of muscular motion, weight, and position.

(4) proprioceptive awareness: the identification of the positions of body parts in space.

(5) ocular control: the localization and visual tracking of stimuli.

(6) vestibular awareness: the detection of motion and gravitational pull as related to one's performance in functional activities, ambulation, and balance.

(7) auditory awareness: the differentiation and identification of sounds.

(8) gustatory awareness: the differentiation and identification of tastes.

(9) olfactory awareness: the differentiation and identification of smells.

b. *Visual–Spatial Awareness*

Visual–spatial awareness refers to skill and performance in perceiving distances between and relationships among objects, including self. This includes but is not limited to:

(1) figure–ground: recognition of forms and objects when presented in a configuration with competing stimuli.

(2) form constancy: recognition of forms and objects as the same when presented in different contexts.

(3) position in space: knowledge of one's position in space relative to other objects.

c. *Body Integration*

Body integration refers to skill and performance in perceiving and regulating the position of various muscles and body parts in relationship to each other during static and movement states. This includes but is not limited to:

(1) *body schema*

Body schema refers to the perception of one's physical self through proprioceptive and interoceptive sensations.

(2) *postural balance*

Postural balance refers to skill and performance in developing and maintaining body posture while sitting, standing, or engaging in activity.

(3) *bilateral motor coordination*

Bilateral motor coordination refers to skill and performance in purpose-

(4) *right-left discrimination*

Right–left discrimination refers to skill and performance in differentiating right from left and vice versa.

(5) *visual–motor integration*

Visual–motor integration refers to skill and performance in combining visual input with purposeful voluntary movement of the hand and other body parts involved in an activity. Visual–motor integration includes eye-hand coordination.

(6) *crossing the midline*

Crossing the midline refers to skill and performance in crossing the vertical midline of the body.

(7) *praxis*

Praxis refers to skill and performance of purposeful movement that involves motor planning.

C. *Cognitive Components*

Cognitive components refer to skill and performance of the mental processes necessary to know or apprehend by understanding. This includes but is not limited to:

1. *Orientation*

Orientation refers to skill and performance in comprehending, defining, and adjusting oneself in an environment with regard to time, place, and person.

2. *Conceptualization/Comprehension*

Conceptualization/comprehension refers to skill and performance in conceiving and understanding concepts or tasks such as color identification, word recognition, sign concepts, sequencing, matching, association, classification, and abstracting. This includes but is not limited to:

a. *Concentration*

Concentration refers to skill and performance in focusing on a designated task or concept.

b. *Attention Span*

Attention span refers to skill and performance in focusing on a task or concept for a particular length of time.

c. *Memory*

Memory refers to skill and performance in retaining and recalling tasks or concepts from the past.

3. *Cognitive Integration*

Cognitive integration refers to skill and performance in applying diverse knowledge to environmental situations. This involves but is not limited to:

a. *Generalization*

Generalization refers to skill and performance in applying specific concepts to a variety of related situations.

b. *Problem Solving*

Problem solving refers to skill and performance in identifying and organizing solutions to difficulties. It includes but is not limited to:

(1) defining or evaluating the problem

(2) organizing a plan

(3) making decisions/judgments

(4) implementing plan, including following through in logical sequence

144

(5) evaluating decision/judgement and plan

D. *Psychosocial Components*

Psychosocial components refer to skill and performance in self–management, dyadic and group interaction.

1. *Self–management*

    Self–management refers to skill and performance in expressing and controlling oneself in functional and creative activities.

    a. *Self–expression*

    Self–expression refers to skill and performance in perceiving one's feelings and interpreting and using a variety of communication signs and symbols. This includes but is not limited to:

    (1) experiencing and recognizing a range of emotions

    (2) having an adequate vocabulary

    (3) having writing and speaking skills

    (4) interpreting and using correctly an adequate range of nonverbal signs and symbols

    b. *Self–control*

    Self–control refers to skill and performance in modulating and modifying present behaviors, and in initiating new behaviors in accordance with situational demands. It includes but is not limited to:

    (1) observing own and others' behavior

    (2) conceptualizing problems in terms of needed behavioral changes or action

    (3) imitating new behaviors

    (4) directing and redirecting energies into stress–reducing activities and behaviors

2. *Dyadic Interaction*

    Dyadic interaction refers to skill and performance in relating to another person. This includes but is not limited to:

    a. understanding social/cultural norms of communication and interaction in various activity and social situations.

    b. setting limits on self and others.

    c. compromising and negotiating.

    d. handling competition, frustration, anxiety, success, and failure.

    e. cooperating and competing with others.

    f. responsibly relying on self and others.

3. *Group Interaction*

    Group interaction refers to skill and performance in relating to groups of three to six persons, or larger. This includes but is not limited to:

    a. knowing and performing a variety of task and social/emotional role behaviors.

    b. understanding common stages of group process.

    c. participating in a group in a manner that is mutually beneficial to self and others.

E. *Therapeutic Adaptations*

Therapeutic adaptations refer to the design and/or restructuring of the physical environment to assist self–care, work, and play/leisure performance. This includes selecting, obtaining, fitting, and fabricating equipment, and instructing the client, family, and/or staff in proper use and care of equipment. It also includes minor repair and modification for correct fit, position, or use. Categories of therapeutic adaptations consist of:

1. *Orthotics*

   Orthotics refer to the provision of dynamic and static splints, braces, and slings for the purpose of relieving pain, maintaining joint alignment, protecting joint integrity, improving function, and/or decreasing deformity.

2. *Prosthetics*

   Prosthetics refer to the training in use of artificial substitutes of missing body parts, which augment performance of function.

3. *Assistive/Adaptive Equipment*

   Assistive/adaptive equipment refers to the provision of special devices that assist in performance, and/or structural or positional changes such as the installation of ramps, bars, changes in furniture heights, adjustments of traffic patterns, and modifications of wheelchairs.

F. *Prevention*

   Prevention refers to skill and performance in minimizing debilitation. It may include programs for persons where predisposition to disability exists, as well as for those who have already incurred a disability. This includes but is not limited to:

   1. *Energy Conservation*

      Energy conservation refers to skill and performance in applying energy–saving procedures, activity restriction, work simplification, time management, and/or organization of the environment to minimize energy output.

   2. *Joint Protection/Body Mechanics*

      Joint protection/body mechanics refers to skill and performance in applying principles or procedures to minimize stress on joints. Procedures may include the use of proper body mechanics, avoidance of static or deforming postures, and/or avoidance of excessive weight bearing.

   3. *Positioning*

      Positioning refers to skill and performance in the placement of a body part in alignment to promote optimal functioning.

   4. *Coordination of Daily Living Activities*

      Coordination of daily living activities refers to skill and performance in selecting and coordinating activities of self–care, work, play/leisure, and rest to promote optimal performance of daily life tasks.

III. *PATIENT/CLIENT–RELATED CONFERENCES*

   Patient/client–related conferences include participating in meetings to discuss and identify needs, treatment program, and future plans of referred client, and documenting such participation. Patient/client may or may not be present. Categories of conferences include:

   A. *Professional Conferences*

      Professional conferences refer to participating in meetings with a group or individual professionals to discuss patient's/client's status, and to advise/consult regarding treatment needs. Synonymous terms for professional conferences include initial conference, interim review, discharge planning, case conference, and others.

   B. *Agency Conferences*

      Agency conferences refer to participating in meetings with vocational, social, religious, recreational, health, educational, and other community representatives to assess, implement, or coordinate the use of services.

   C. *Client–Advocate Conferences*

Client–advocate conferences refer to participating in meetings with client advocate (e.g., family, guardian, or others responsible for patient/client) to assess patient's/client's situation, set goals, plan treatment and/or discharge; and/or to instruct client advocate to support or carry out treatment program.

IV. TRAVEL: PATIENT–TREATMENT RELATED

Travel: patient–treatment related refers to travel by therapists, with or without patient; that is, related to direct patient treatment.

Appendix C

UNIFORM TERMINOLOGY FOR REPORTING OCCUPATIONAL THERAPY SERVICES,
SECOND EDITION

Used by permission of the American Occupational Therapy Association, Inc., Rockville, Maryland.

Uniform Terminology for Occupational Therapy—Second Edition delineates and defines Occupational Performance Areas and Occupational Performance Components that are addressed in occupational therapy direct service. These definitions are provided to facilitate the uniform use of terminology and definitions throughout the profession. The original document, *Occupational Therapy Product Output Reporting System and Uniform Terminology for Reporting Occupational Therapy Services*, which was published in 1979, helped create a base of consistent terminology that was used in many of the official documents of The American Occupational Therapy Association, Inc. (AOTA), in occupational therapy education curricula, and in a variety of occupational therapy practice settings. In order to remain current with practice, the first document was revised over a period of several years with extensive feedback from the profession. The revisions were completed in 1988. It is recognized and recommended that a document of this nature be updated periodically so that occupational therapy is defined in accordance with current theory and practice.

Guidelines for Use

Uniform Terminology—Second Edition may be used in a variety of ways. It defines occupational therapy practice, which includes occupational performance areas and occupational performance components. In addition, it will be useful to occupational therapists for (a) documentation, (b) charge systems, (c) education, (d) program development, (e) marketing, and (f) research. Examples of how *Occupational Performance Areas* and *Occupational Performance Components* translate into practice are provided below. It is not the intent of this document to define specific occupational therapy programs nor specific occupational therapy interventions. Some examples of the differences between occupational performance areas and occupational performance components and programs and interventions are:

1. An individual who is injured on the job may be able to return to work, which is an occupational performance area. In order to achieve the outcome of returning to work, the individual may need to address specific performance components such as strength, endurance, and time management. The occupational therapist, in cooperation with the vocational team, utilizes planned interventions to achieve the desired outcome. These interventions may include activities such as an exercise program, body mechanics instruction, and job modification, and may be provided in a work-hardening program.

2. An individual with severe physical limitations may need and desire the opportunity to live within a community-integrated setting, which represents the *Occupational Performance Areas* of activities of daily living and work. In order to achieve the outcome of community living, the individual may need to address specific *Performance Components*, such as normalizing muscle tone, gross motor coordination, postural control, and self-management. The occupational therapist, in cooperation with the team, utilizes planned interventions to achieve the desired outcome. Interventions may include neuromuscular facilitation, object manipulation, instruction in use of adaptive equipment, use of environmental control systems, and functional positioning for eating. These interventions may be provided in a community-based independent living program.

3. A child with learning disabilities may need to perform educational activities within a public school setting. Since learning is a student's work, this educational activity would be considered the *Occupational Performance Area* for this individual. In order to achieve the educational outcome of efficient and effective completion of written classroom work, the child may need to address specific *Occupational Performance Components*, including sensory processing, perceptual skills, postural control, and motor skills. The occupational therapist, in cooperation with the team, utilizes planned interventions to achieve the desired outcome. Interventions may include activities such as adapting the student's seating to improve postural control and stability and practicing motor control and coordination. This program could be provided by school district personnel or through contract services.

4. An infant with cerebral palsy may need to participate in developmental activities to engage in the *Occupational Performance Areas* of activities of daily living and play. The developmental outcomes may be achieved by addressing specific *Performance Components* such as sensory awareness and neuromuscular control. The occupational therapist, in cooperation with the team, utilizes planned interventions to achieve the desired outcomes. Interventions may include activities such as seating and positioning for play, neuromuscular facilitation techniques to enable eating,

and parent training. These interventions may be provided in a home-based occupational therapy program.

5. An adult with schizophrenia may need and desire to live independently in the community, which represents the *Occupational Performance Areas* of activities of daily living, work activities, and play or leisure activities. The specific *Occupational Performance Areas* may be medication routine, functional mobility, home management, vocational exploration, play or leisure performance, and social skills. In order to achieve the outcome of living alone, the individual may need to address specific performance components such as topographical orientation, memory, categorization, problem solving, interests, social conduct, and time management. The occupational therapist, in cooperation with the team, utilizes planned interventions to achieve the desired outcome. Interventions may include activities such as training in the use of public transportation, instruction in budgeting skills, selection of and participation in social activities, and instruction in social conduct. These interventions may be provided in a community-based mental health program.

6. An individual who abuses substances may need to reestablish family roles and responsibilities, which represents the *Occupational Performance Areas* of activities of daily living and work. In order to achieve the outcome of family participation, the individual may need to address the *Performance Components* of roles, values, social conduct, self-expression, coping skills, and self-control. The occupational therapist, in cooperation with the team, utilizes planned intervention to achieve the desired outcomes. Interventions may include role and value clarification exercises, role-playing, instruction in stress management techniques, and parenting skills. These interventions may be provided in an inpatient acute care unit.

Because of the extensive use of the original document (*Uniform Terminology for Reporting Occupational Therapy Services, 1979*) in official documents, this revision is a second edition and does not completely replace the 1979 version. This follows the practice that other professions, such as medicine, pursue with their documents. Examples are the *Physician's Current Procedural Terminology First—Fourth Editions (CPT 1-4)* and the *Diagnostic and Statistical Manual First—Third Editions (DSM-I-III-R)*. Therefore, this document is presented as *Uniform Terminology for Occupational Therapy, — Second Edition*.

Background

Task Force Charge. In 1983, the Representative Assembly of the American Occupational Therapy Association charged the Commission on Practice to form a task force to revise the *Occupational Therapy Product Output Reporting System and Uniform Terminology for Reporting Occupational Therapy Services*. The document had been approved by the Representative Assembly in 1979 and needed to be updated to reflect current practice.

Background Information

The *Occupational Therapy Product Output Reporting System and Uniform Terminology for Reporting Occupational Therapy Services* (hereafter to be referred to as *Product Output Reporting System* or *Uniform Terminology*) document was originally developed in response to the Medicare-Medicaid Anti-Fraud and Abuse Amendments of 1977 (Public Law 95-142), which required the Secretary of the Department of Health and Human Services to establish regulations for uniform reporting systems for all departments in hospitals. The AOTA developed the documents to create a uniform reporting system for occupational therapy departments. Although the Department of Health and Human Services never adopted the system because of antitrust concerns relating to price fixing, occupational therapists have used the documents extensively in the profession.

Three states, Maryland, California, and Washington, have used the *Product Output Reporting System* as a basis for statewide reporting systems. AOTA's official documents have relied on the definitions to create uniformity. Many occupational therapy schools and departments have used the definitions to guide education and documentation. Although the initial need was for reimbursement reporting systems, the profession has used the documents primarily to facilitate uniformity in definitions.

Task Force Formation

In 1983, Linda Kohlman McGourty, a member of the AOTA Commission on Practice, was appointed by the commission's chair, John Farace, to chair the Uniform Terminology Task Force. Initially, a notice was placed in the *Occupational Therapy Newspaper* for people to submit feedback for the revisions. Many responses were received. Before the task force was appointed in 1984, Maryland, California, and Washington adopted reimbursement systems based on the *Product Output Reporting System*. Therefore, to increase the quantity and quality of input for the revisions, it was decided to postpone the formation of the task force until these states had had an opportunity to use the systems.

In 1985, a second notice was placed in the *Occupational Therapy News* requesting feedback, and a task force was appointed. The following people were selected to serve on the task force:

- Linda Kohlman-McGourty, MOT, OTR, Washington (Chair)
- Roger Smith, MOT, OTR, Wisconsin
- Jane Marvin, OTC, California
- Nancy Mahon Smith, MBA, OTR, Maryland and Arkansas
- Mary Foto, OTR, California

These people were selected based on the following criteria:

1. Geographical representation
2. Professional expertise
3. Participation in other current AOTA projects
4. Knowledge of reimbursement systems
5. Interest in serving on the task force

Development of the Uniform Terminology, — Second Edition. The task force met in 1986 and 1987 to develop drafts of the revisions. A draft from the task force was submitted to the Commission on Practice in May of 1987. Listed below are several decisions that were made in the revision process by the task force and the Commission on Practice.

1. To not replace the original document (*Uniform Terminology for Reporting Occupational Therapy Services, 1979*) because of the number of official documents based on it and the need to retain a *Product Output Reporting System* as an official document of the AOTA.
2. To limit the revised document to defining occupational performance areas and occupational performance components for occupational therapy intervention (i.e.,

indirect services were deleted and the *Product Output Reporting System* was not revised) to make the project manageable.

3. To coordinate the revision process with other current AOTA projects such as the Professional and Technical Role Analysis (PATRA) and the Occupational Therapy Comprehensive Functional Assessment of the American Occupational Therapy Foundation (AOTF).

4. To develop a document that reflects current areas of practice and facilitates uniformity of definitions in the profession.

5. To recommend that the AOTA develop a companion document to define techniques, modalities, and activities used in occupational therapy intervention and a document to define specific programs that are offered by occupational therapy departments. The Commission on Practice subsequently developed educational materials to assist in the application of uniform terminology to practice.

Several drafts of the revised *Uniform Terminology, Second Edition* document were reviewed by appropriate AOTA commissions and committees and by a selected review network based on geographical representation, professional expertise, and demonstrated leadership in the field. Excellent responses were received, and the feedback was incorporated into the final document by the Commission on Practice.

Occupational Therapy Assessment

Occupational Therapy Intervention

I. Occupational Therapy Performance Areas
   A. Activities of Daily Living
      1. Grooming
      2. Oral Hygiene
      3. Bathing
      4. Toilet Hygiene
      5. Dressing
      6. Feeding and Eating
      7. Medication Routine
      8. Socialization
      9. Functional Communication
      10. Functional Mobility
      11. Sexual Expression
   B. Work Activities
      1. Home Management
         a. Clothing Care
         b. Cleaning
         c. Meal Preparation and Cleanup
         d. Shopping
         e. Money Management
         f. Household Maintenance
         g. Safety Procedures
      2. Care of Others
      3. Educational Activities

        4. Vocational Activities
            a. Vocational Exploration
            b. Job Acquisition
            c. Work or Job Performance
            d. Retirement Planning
    C. Play or Leisure Activities
        1. Play or Leisure Exploration
        2. Play or Leisure Performance
II. Performance Components
    A. Sensory Motor Component
        1. Sensory Integration
            a. Sensory Awareness
            b. Sensory Processing
                (1) tactile
                (2) proprioceptive
                (3) vestibular
                (4) visual
                (5) auditory
                (6) gustatory
                (7) olfactory
            c. Perceptual Skills
                (1) stereognosis
                (2) kinesthesia
                (3) body scheme
                (4) right-left discrimination
                (5) form constancy
                (6) position in space
                (7) visual closure
                (8) figure-ground
                (9) depth perception
                (10) topographical orientation
        2. Neuromuscular
            a. Reflex
            b. Range of Motion
            c. Muscle Tone
            d. Strength
            e. Endurance
            f. Postural Control
            g. Soft Tissue Integrity
        3. Motor
            a. Activity Tolerance
            b. Gross Motor Coordination
            c. Crossing the Midline
            d. Laterality
            e. Bilateral Integration
            f. Praxis
            g. Fine Motor Coordination/Dexterity
            h. Visual-Motor Integration
            i. Oral-Motor Control

B. Cognitive Integration and Cognitive Components
   1. Level of Arousal
   2. Orientation
   3. Recognition
   4. Attention Span
   5. Memory
      a. Short-Term
      b. Long-Term
      c. Remote
      d. Recent
   6. Sequencing
   7. Categorization
   8. Concept Formation
   9. Intellectual Operations in Space
   10. Problem Solving
   11. Generalization of Learning
   12. Integration of Learning
   13. Synthesis of Learning
C. Psychosocial Skills and Psychological Components
   1. Psychological
      a. Roles
      b. Values
      c. Interests
      d. Initiation of Activity
      e. Termination of Activity
      f. Self-Concept
   2. Social
      a. Social Conduct
      b. Conversation
      c. Self-Expression
   3. Self-Management
      a. Coping Skills
      b. Time Management
      c. Self-Control

Occupational Therapy Assessment

Assessment is the planned process of obtaining, interpreting, and documenting the functional status of the individual. The purpose of the assessment is to identify the individual's abilities and limitations, including deficits, delays, or maladaptive behavior that can be addressed in occupational therapy intervention. Data can be gathered through a review of records, observation, interview, and the administration of test procedures. Such procedures include, but are not limited to, the use of standardized tests, questionnaires, performance checklists, activities, and tasks designed to evaluate specific performance abilities.

Occupational Therapy Intervention

Occupational therapy addresses function and uses specific procedures and activities to (a) develop, maintain, improve, and/or restore the performance of necessary functions; (b) compensate for dysfunction; (c) minimize or prevent debilitation; and/or (d) promote health and wellness. Categories of function are defined as occupational performance areas and performance components. Occupational performance areas include activities of daily living, work activities, and play/leisure activities. Performance components refer to the functional abilities required for occupational performance, including sensory motor, cognitive, and psychological components. Deficits or delays in these occupational performance areas may be addressed by occupational therapy intervention.

I. Occupational Performance Areas
  A. Activities of Daily Living
    1. *Grooming:* Obtain and use supplies to shave; apply and remove cosmetics; wash, comb, style, and brush hair; care for nails; care for skin; and apply deodorant.
    2. *Oral Hygiene:* Obtain and use supplies; clean mouth and teeth; remove, clean and reinsert dentures.
    3. *Bathing:* Obtain and use supplies; soap, rinse, and dry all body parts; maintain bathing position; transfer to and from bathing position.
    4. *Toilet Hygiene:* Obtain and use supplies; clean self; transfer to and from, and maintain toileting position on, bedpan, toilet, or commode.
    5. *Dressing:* Select appropriate clothing; obtain clothing from storage area; dress and undress in a sequential fashion; and fasten and adjust clothing and shoes. Don and doff assistive or adaptive equipment, prostheses, or orthoses.
    6. *Feeding and Eating:* Set up food; use appropriate utensils and tableware; bring food or drink to mouth; suck, masticate, cough, and swallow.
    7. *Medication Routine:* Obtain medication; open and close containers; and take prescribed quantities as scheduled.
    8. *Socialization:* Interact in appropriate contextual and cultural ways.
    9. *Functional Communication:* Use equipment or systems to enhance or provide communication, such as writing equipment, telephones, typewriters, communication boards, call lights, emergency systems, braille writers, augmentative communication systems, and computers.
    10. *Functional Mobility:* Move from one position or place to another, such as in bed mobility, wheelchair mobility, transfers (bed, car, tub, toilet, chair), and functional ambulation, with or without use of adaptive aids, driving, and use of public transportation.
    11. *Sexual Expression:* Recognize, communicate, and perform desired sexual activities.
  B. Work Activities
    1. *Home Management*
      a. Clothing Care: Obtain and use supplies, launder, iron, store, and mend.
      b. Cleaning: Obtain and use supplies, pick up, vacuum, sweep, dust, scrub, mop, make bed, and remove trash.
      c. Meal Preparation and Cleanup: Plan nutritious meals and prepare food; open and close containers, cabinets, and drawers; use kitchen utensils and appliances; and clean up and store food.

    d. Shopping: Select and purchase items and perform money transactions.

    e. Money Management: Budget, pay bills, and use bank systems.

    f. Household Maintenance: Maintain home, yard, garden appliances, and household items, and/or obtain appropriate assistance.

    g. Safety Procedures: Know and perform prevention and emergency procedures to maintain a safe environment and prevent injuries.

2. *Care of Others:* Provide for children, spouse, parents, or others, such as the physical care, nurturance, communication, and use of age-appropriate activities.

3. *Educational Activities:* Participate in a school environment and school-sponsored activities (such as field trips, work-study, and extracurricular activities).

4. *Vocational Activities*

    a. Vocational Exploration: Determine aptitudes, interests, skills, and appropriate vocational pursuits.

    b. Job Acquisition: Identify and select work opportunities and complete application and interview processes.

    c. Work of Job Performance: Perform job tasks in a timely and effective manner, incorporating necessary work behaviors such as grooming, interpersonal skills, punctuality, and adherence to safety procedures.

    d. Retirement Planning: Determine aptitudes, interests, skills, and identify appropriate avocational pursuits.

C. Play or Leisure Activities

1. *Play or Leisure Exploration:* Identify interests, skills, opportunities, and appropriate play or leisure activities.

2. *Play or Leisure Performance:* Participate in play or leisure activities, using physical and psychosocial skills.

    a. Maintain a balance of play or leisure activities with work and activities of daily living.

    b. Obtain, utilize, and maintain equipment and supplies.

II. Performance Components

A. Sensory Motor Component

1. *Sensory Integration*

    a. Sensory Awareness: Receive and differentiate sensory stimuli.

    b. Sensory Processing: Interpret sensory stimuli.

      (1) Tactile: Interpret light touch, pressure, temperature, pain, vibration, and two-point stimuli through skin contact/receptors.

      (2) Proprioceptive: Interpret stimuli originating in muscles, joints, and other internal tissues to give information about the position of one body part in relationship to another.

      (3) Vestibular: Interpret stimuli from the inner ear receptors regarding head position and movement.

      (4) Visual: Interpret stimuli through the eyes, including peripheral vision and acuity, awareness of color, depth, and figure-ground.

      (5) Auditory: Interpret sounds, localize sounds, and discriminate background sounds.

      (6) Gustatory: Interpret tastes.

      (7) Olfactory: Interpret odors.

    c. Perceptual Skills

      (1) Stereognosis: Identify objects through the sense of touch.

(2) Kinesthesia: Identify the excursion and direction of joint movement.

(3) Body Schema: Acquire an internal awareness of the body and the relationship of body parts to each other.

(4) Right-Left Discrimination: Differentiate one side of the body from the other.

(5) Form Constancy: Recognize forms and objects as the same in various environments, positions, and sizes.

(6) Position in Space: Determine the spatial relationship of figures and objects to self or other forms and objects.

(7) Visual Closure: Identify forms or objects from incomplete presentations.

(8) Figure-Ground: Differentiate between foreground and background forms and objects.

(9) Depth Perception: Determine the relative distance between objects, figures, or landmarks and the observer.

(10) Topographical Orientation: Determine the location of objects and settings and the route to the location.

2. *Neuromuscular*
   a. Reflex: Present an involuntary muscle response elicited by sensory input.
   b. Range of Motion: Move body parts through an arc.
   c. Muscle Tone: Demonstrate a degree of tension or resistance in a muscle.
   d. Strength: Demonstrate a degree of muscle power when movement is resisted as with weight or gravity.
   e. Endurance: Sustain cardiac, pulmonary, and musculoskeletal exertion over time.
   f. Postural Control: Position and maintain head, neck, trunk, and limb alignment with appropriate weight shifting, midline orientation, and righting reactions for function.
   g. Soft Tissue Integrity: Maintain anatomical and physiological condition of interstitial tissue and skin.

3. *Motor*
   a. Activity Tolerance: Sustain a purposeful activity over time.
   b. Gross Motor Coordination: Use large muscle groups for controlled movements.
   c. Crossing the Midline: Move limbs and eyes across the sagittal plane of the body.
   d. Laterality: Use a preferred unilateral body part for activities requiring a high level of skill.
   e. Bilateral Integration: Interact with both body sides in a coordinated manner during activity.
   f. Praxis: Conceive and plan a new motor act in response to an environmental demand.
   g. Fine Motor Coordination/Dexterity: Use small muscle groups for controlled movements, particularly in object manipulation.
   h. Visual-Motor Integration: Coordinate the interaction of visual information with body movement during activity.
   i. Oral-Motor Control: Coordinate oro-pharyngeal musculature for controlled movements.

B. Cognitive Integration and Cognitive Components
   1. *Level of Arousal:* Demonstrate alertness and responsiveness to environ-

mental stimuli.

2. *Orientation:* Identify person, place, time, and situation.
3. *Recognition:* Identify familiar faces, objects, and other previously presented materials.
4. *Attention Span:* Focus on a task over time.
5. *Memory*
   a. Short-Term: Recall information for brief periods of time.
   b. Long-Term: Recall information for long periods of time.
   c. Remote: Recall events from distant past.
   d. Recent: Recall events from immediate past.
6. *Sequencing:* Place information, concepts, and actions in order.
7. *Categorization:* Identify similarities of and differences between environmental information.
8. *Concept Formation:* Organize a variety of information to form thoughts and ideas.
9. *Intellectual Operations in Space:* Mentally manipulate spatial relationships.
10. *Problem Solving:* Recognize a problem, define a problem, identify alternative plans, select a plan, organize steps in a plan, implement a plan, and evaluate the outcome.
11. *Generalization of Learning:* Apply previously learned concepts and behaviors to similar situations.
12. *Integration of Learning:* Incorporate previously acquired concepts and behavior into a variety of new situations.
13. *Synthesis of Learning:* Restructure previously learned concepts and behaviors into new patterns.

C. Psychosocial Skills and Psychological Components
1. *Psychological*
   a. Roles: Identify functions one assumes or acquires in society (e.g., worker, student, parent, church member).
   b. Values: Identify ideas or beliefs that are intrinsically important.
   c. Interests: Identify mental or physical activities that create pleasure and maintain attention.
   d. Initiation of Activity: Engage in a physical or mental activity.
   e. Termination of Activity: Stop an activity at an appropriate time.
   f. Self-Concept: Develop value of physical and emotional self.
2. *Social*
   a. Social Conduct: Interact using manners, personal space, eye contact, gestures, active listening, and self-expression appropriate to one's environment.
   b. Conversation: Use verbal and nonverbal communication to interact in a variety of settings.
   c. Self-Expression: Use a variety of styles and skills to express thoughts, feelings, and needs.
3. *Self-Management*
   a. Coping Skills: Identify and manage stress and related reactors.
   b. Time Management: Plan and participate in a balance of self-care, work, leisure, and rest activities to promote satisfaction and health.
   c. Self-Control: Modulate and modify one's own behavior in response to environmental needs, demands, and constraints.

References

American Medical Association. (1966-1988). *Physicians' current procedural terminology, first-fourth editions.* Chicago: Author.

American Occupational Therapy Association. (1979). *Occupational therapy output reporting system and uniform terminology for reporting occupational therapy services.* Rockville, MD: Author.

American Psychiatric Association. (1952-1987). *Diagnostic and statistical manual of mental disorders first-third editions (DSM-I-III-R)* Washington, DC: Author.

Medicare-Medicaid Anti-Fraud and Abuse Amendments (Public Law 95-142). (1977). 42 U.S.C. § 1305.

Prepared by the Uniform Terminology Task Force (Linda Kohlman McGourty, MOT OTR, Chair, and Mary Foto, OTR, Jane K. Marvin, MA, OTC, CIRS, Nancy Mahan Smith, MBA, OTR, and Roger O. Smith, MOT, OTR, task force members) and members of the Commission on Practice, with contributions from Susan Kronsnoble, OTR, for the Commission on Practice (L. Randy Strickland, EdD, OTR, FAOTA, Chair). Approved by the Representative Assembly April 1989.

Figures C-1, C-2, and C-3 are flow charts created by the authors to aid in the interpretation of treatment based on Uniform Terminology, Second Edition.

OCCUPATIONAL PERFORMANCE

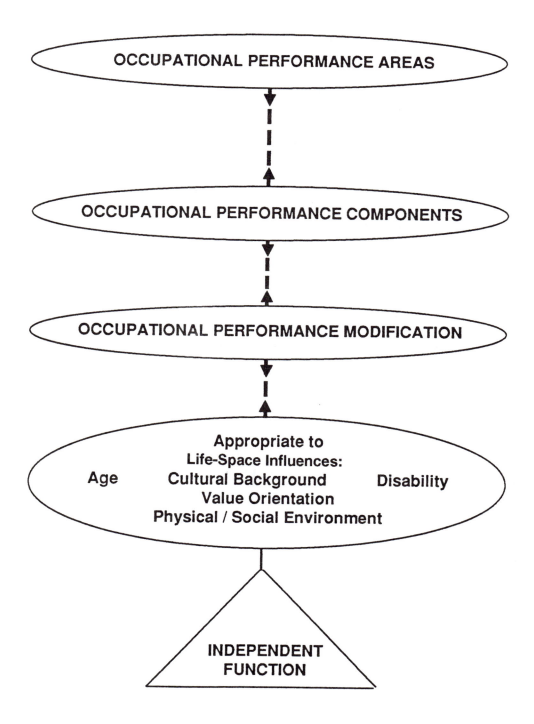

Figure C-1.

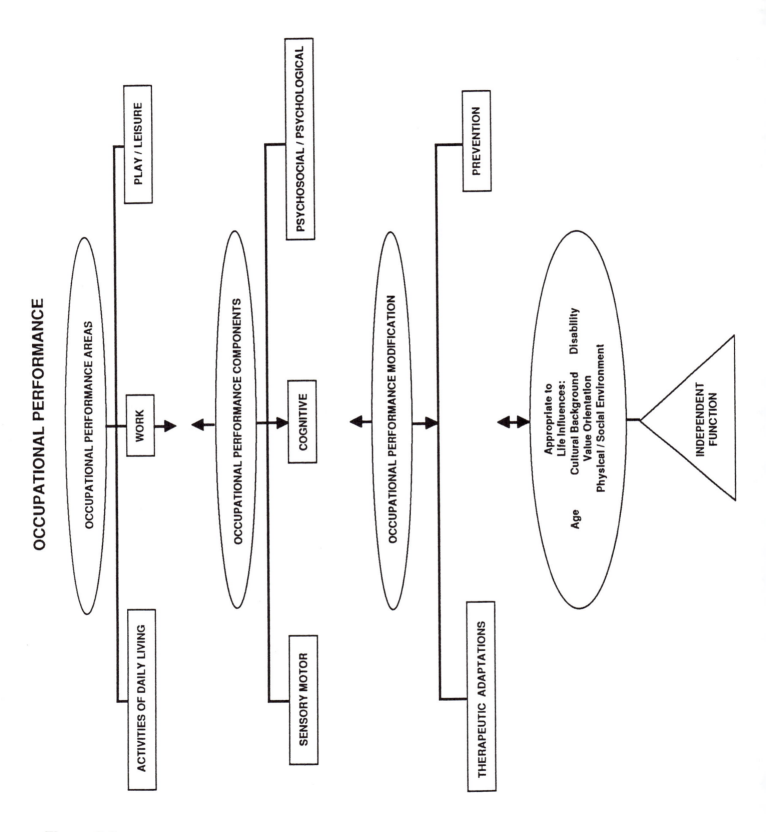

Figure C-2.

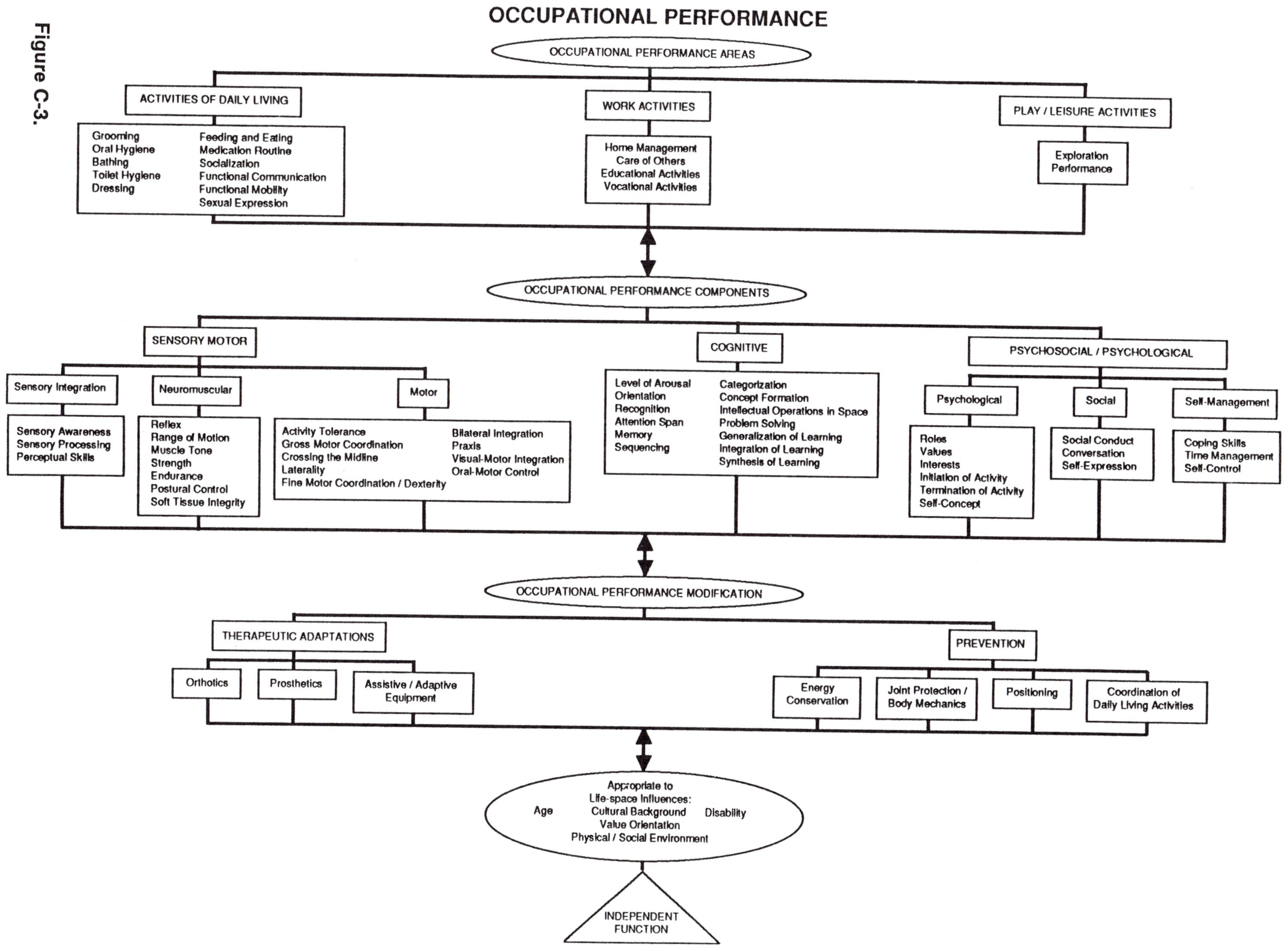

OCCUPATIONAL PERFORMANCE

OCCUPATIONAL PERFORMANCE AREAS

ACTIVITIES OF DAILY LIVING

Grooming
Oral Hygiene
Bathing
Toilet Hygiene
Dressing

Feeding and Eating
Medication Routine
Socialization
Functional Communication
Functional Mobility
Sexual Expression

WORK ACTIVITIES

Home Management
Care of Others
Educational Activities
Vocational Activities

PLAY / LEISURE ACTIVITIES

Exploration
Performance

OCCUPATIONAL PERFORMANCE COMPONENTS

SENSORY MOTOR

Sensory Integration

Sensory Awareness
Sensory Processing
Perceptual Skills

Neuromuscular

Reflex
Range of Motion
Muscle Tone
Strength
Endurance
Postural Control
Soft Tissue Integrity

Motor

Activity Tolerance
Gross Motor Coordination
Crossing the Midline
Laterality
Fine Motor Coordination / Dexterity

Bilateral Integration
Praxis
Visual-Motor Integration
Oral-Motor Control

COGNITIVE

Level of Arousal
Orientation
Recognition
Attention Span
Memory
Sequencing

Categorization
Concept Formation
Intellectual Operations in Space
Problem Solving
Generalization of Learning
Integration of Learning
Synthesis of Learning

PSYCHOSOCIAL / PSYCHOLOGICAL

Psychological

Roles
Values
Interests
Initiation of Activity
Termination of Activity
Self-Concept

Social

Social Conduct
Conversation
Self-Expression

Self-Management

Coping Skills
Time Management
Self-Control

OCCUPATIONAL PERFORMANCE MODIFICATION

THERAPEUTIC ADAPTATIONS

Orthotics

Prosthetics

Assistive / Adaptive Equipment

PREVENTION

Energy Conservation

Joint Protection / Body Mechanics

Positioning

Coordination of Daily Living Activities

Appropriate to

Age

Life-space Influences:
Cultural Background
Value Orientation
Physical / Social Environment

Disability

INDEPENDENT FUNCTION

Figure C-3.

Appendix D

UNIFORM TERMINOLOGY FOR REPORTING OCCUPATIONAL THERAPY SERVICES,
THIRD EDITION

Used by permission of The American Occupational Therapy Association, Inc., Rockville, Maryland

This is an official document of The American Occupational Therapy Association. This document is intended to provide a generic outline of the domain of concern of occupational therapy and is designed to create common terminology for the profession and to capture the essence of occupational therapy succinctly for others.

It is recognized that the phenomena that constitute the profession's domain of concern can be categorized, and labeled, in a number of different ways. This document is not meant to limit those in the field, formulating theories or frames of reference, who may wish to combine or refine particular constructs. It is also not meant to limit those who would like to conceptualize the profession's domain of concern in a different manner.

Introduction

The first edition of Uniform Terminology was approved and published in 1979 (AOTA, 1979). In 1989, the *Uniform Terminology for Occupational Therapy—Second Edition* (AOTA, 1989) was approved and published. The second document presented an organized structure for understanding the areas of practice for the profession of occupational therapy. The document outlined two domains. **PERFORMANCE AREAS** (activities of daily living [ADL], work and productive activities, and play or leisure) include activities that the occupational therapy practitioner[1] emphasizes when determining functional abilities. **PERFORMANCE COMPONENTS** (sensorimotor, cognitive, psychosocial, and psychological aspects) are the elements of performance that occupational therapists assess and, when needed, in which they intervene for improved performance.

This third edition has been further expanded to reflect current practice and to incorporate contextual aspects of performance. *Performance Areas, Performance Components,* and *Performance Contexts* are the parameters of occupational therapy's domain of concern. *Performance areas* are broad categories of human activity that are typically part of daily life. They are activities of daily living, work and productive activities, and play or leisure activities. *Performance components* are fundamental human abilities that—to varying degrees and in differing combinations—are required for successful engagement in performance areas.

These components are sensorimotor, cognitive, psychosocial, and psychological. *Performance contexts* are situations or factors that influence an individual's engagement in desired and/or required performance areas. Performance contexts consist of *temporal* aspects (chronological age, developmental age, place in life cycle, and health status) and *environmental* aspects (physical, social, and cultural considerations). There is an interactive relationship among performance areas, performance components, and performance contexts. Function in performance areas is the ultimate concern of occupational therapy, with performance components considered as they relate to participation in performance areas. Performance areas and performance components are always viewed within performance contexts. Performance contexts are taken into consideration when determining function and dysfunction relative to performance areas and performance components, and in planning intervention. For example, the occupational therapist does not evaluate strength (a performance component) in isolation. Strength is considered as it affects necessary or desired tasks (performance areas). If the individual is interested in homemaking, the occupational therapy practitioner would consider the interaction of strength with homemaking tasks. Strengthening could be addressed through kitchen activities, such as cooking and putting groceries away. In some cases, the practitioner would employ an adaptive approach and recommend that the family switch from heavy stoneware to lighter-weight dishes, or use lighter-weight pots on the stove to enable the individual to make dinner safely without becoming fatigued or compromising safety.

Occupational therapy assessment involves examining performance areas, performance components, and performance contexts. Intervention may be directed toward elements of performance areas (e.g., dressing, vocational exploration), performance components (e.g., endurance, problem solving), or the environmental aspects of performance contexts. In the last case, the physical and/or social environment may be altered or augmented to improve and/or maintain function. After identifying the performance areas the individual wishes or needs to address, the occupational therapist assesses the features of the environments in which the talks will be performed. If an individual's job requires cooking in a restaurant as opposed to leisure cooking at home, the occupational therapy practitioner faces several challenges to enable the individual's success in different environments. Therefore, the third critical aspect of performance is the performance context, the features of the environment

166

that affect the person's ability to engage in functional activities.

This document categorizes specific activities in each of the performance areas (ADL, work and productive activities, play or leisure). This categorization is based on what is considered "typical," and is not meant to imply that a particular individual characterizes personal activities in the same manner as someone else. Occupational therapy practitioners embrace individual differences, and so would document the unique pattern of the individual being served, rather than forcing the "typical" pattern on him or her and family. For example, because of experience or culture, a particular individual might think of home management as an ADL task rather than "work and productive activities" (current listing). Socialization might be considered part of play or leisure activity instead of its current listing as part of "activities of daily living," because of life experience or cultural heritage.

Examples in Practice

Uniform Terminology—Third Edition defines occupational therapy's domain of concern, which includes performance areas, performance components, and performance contexts. While this document may be used by occupational therapy practitioners in a number of different areas (e.g., practice, documentation, charge systems, education, program development, marketing, research, disability classifications, and regulations), it focuses on the use of uniform terminology in practice. This document is not intended to define specific occupational therapy interventions. Examples of how performance areas, performance components, and performance contexts translate into practice are provided below.

- An individual who is injured on the job may have the potential to return to work and productive activities, which is a performance area. In order to achieve the outcome of returning to work and productive activities, the individual may need to address specific performance components such as strength, endurance, soft tissue integrity, time management, and the physical features of performance contexts, like structures and objects in his or her environment. The occupational therapy practitioner, in collaboration with the individual and other members of the vocational team, uses planned interventions to achieve the desired outcome. These interventions may include activities such as an exercise program, body mechanics instruction, and job site modifications, all of which may be provided in a work-hardening program.

- An elderly individual recovering from a cerebral vascular accident may wish to live in a community setting, which combines the performance areas of ADL with work and productive activities. In order to achieve the outcome of community living, the individual may need to address specific performance components, such as muscle tone, gross motor coordination, postural control, and self-management. It is also necessary to consider the sociocultural and physical features of performance contexts, such as support available from other persons, and adaptations of structures and objects within the environment. The occupational therapy practitioner, in cooperation with the team, utilizes planned interventions to achieve the desired outcome. Interventions may include neuromuscular facilitation, practice of object manipulation, and instruction in the use of adaptive equipment and home safety equipment. The practitioner and individual also pursue the selection and training of a personal assistant to ensure the completion of ADL tasks. These interventions may be provided in a comprehensive inpatient rehabilitation unit.

- A child with learning disabilities is required to perform educational activities within a public school setting. Engaging in educational activities is considered the performance area of work and productive activities for this child. To achieve the educational outcome of efficient and effective completion of written classroom work, the child may need to address specific performance components. These include sensory processing, perceptual skills, postural control, motor skills, and the physical features of performance contexts, such as objects (e.g., desk, chair) in the environment. In cooperation with the team, occupational therapy interventions may include activities like adapting the student's seating in the classroom to improve postural control and stability, and practicing motor control and coordination. This program could be developed by an occupational therapist and supported by school district personnel.

- The parents of an infant with cerebral palsy may ask to facilitate the child's involvement in the performance areas of activities of daily living and play. Subsequent to assessment, the therapist identifies specific performance components, such as sensory awareness and neuromuscular control. The practitioner also addresses the physical and cultural features of performance contexts. In collaboration with the parents, occupational therapy interventions may include activities such as seating and positioning for play, neuromuscular facilitation techniques to enable eating, facilitating parent skills in caring for and playing with their infant, and modifying the play space for accessibility. These interventions may be provided in a home-based occupational therapy program.

- An adult with schizophrenia may need and want to live independently in the community, which represents the performance areas of activities of daily living, work and productive activities, and leisure activities. The specific performance categories may be medication routine, functional mobility, home management, vocational exploration, play or leisure performance, and social interaction. In order to achieve the outcome of living independently, the individual may need to address specific performance components such as topographical orientation, memory, categorization, problem solving, interests, social conduct, time management, and sociocultural features of performance contexts, such as social factors (e.g., influence of family and friends) and roles. The occupational therapy practitioner, in cooperation with the team, utilizes planned interventions to achieve the desired outcome. Interventions may include activities such as training in the use of public transportation, instruction in budgeting skills, selection of and participation in social activities, and instruction in social conduct. These interventions may be provided in a community-based mental health program.

- An individual with a history of substance abuse may need to reestablish family roles and responsibilities, which represent the performance areas of activities of daily living, work and productive activities, and leisure activities. In order to achieve the outcome of family participation, the individual may need to address the performance components of roles, values, social conduct, self-expression, coping skills, self-control, and the sociocultural features of performance contexts, such as custom, behavior, rules, and rituals. The occupational therapy practitioner, in cooperation with the team, utilizes planned intervention to achieve the desired outcomes. Interventions may include roles and values exercises, instruction in stress management techniques, identification of family roles and activities, and support to develop family leisure routines. These interventions may be provided in an inpatient acute care unit.

Person-Activity-Environment Fit

Person-activity-environment fit refers to the match among skills and abilities of the individual; the demands of the activity; and the characteristics of the physical, social, and cultural environments. It is the interaction among the performance areas, performance components, and performance contexts that is important and determines the success of the performance. When occupational therapy practitioners provide services, they attend to all of these aspects of performance and the interaction among them. They also attend to each individual's unique personal history. The personal history includes one's skills and abilities (performance components), the past performance of specific life tasks (performance areas), and experience within particular environments (performance contexts). In addition to personal history, anticipated life tasks and role demands influence performance.

When considering the person-activity-environment fit, variables such as novelty, importance, motivation, activity tolerance, and quality are salient. Situations range from those that are completely familiar, to those that are novel and have never been experienced. Both the novelty and familiarity within a situation contribute to the overall task performance. In each situation, there is an optimal level of novelty that engages the individual sufficiently and provides enough information to perform the task. When too little novelty is present, the individual may miss cues and opportunities to perform. When too much novelty is present, the individual may become confused and distracted, inhibiting effective task performance.

Humans determine that some stimuli and situations are more meaningful than others. Individuals perform tasks they deem important. It is critical to identify what the individual wants or needs to do when planning interventions.

The level of motivation an individual demonstrates to perform a particular task is determined by both internal and external factors. An individual's biobehavioral state (e.g., amount of rest, arousal, tension) contributes to the potential to be responsive. The features of the social and physical environments (e.g., persons in the room, noise level) provide information that is either adequate or inadequate to produce a motivated state.

Activity tolerance is the individual's ability to sustain a purposeful activity over time. Individuals must not only select, initiate, and terminate activities, but they must also attend to a task for the needed length of time to complete the task and accomplish their goals.

The quality of performance is measured by standards generated by both the individual and others in the social and cultural environments in which the performance occurs. Quality is a continuum of expectations set within particular activities and contexts.

I. Performance Areas
    A. Activities of Daily Living
        1. Grooming
        2. Oral Hygiene
        3. Bathing/Showering
        4. Toilet Hygiene
        5. Personal Device Care
        6. Dressing
        7. Feeding and Eating
        8. Medication Routine
        9. Health Maintenance
      10. Socialization
      11. Functional Communication
      12. Functional Mobility
      13. Community Mobility
      14. Emergency Response

15. Sexual Expression
B. Work and Productive Activities
  1. Home Management
    a. Clothing Care
    b. Cleaning
    c. Meal Preparation/Cleanup
    d. Shopping
    e. Money Management
    f. Household Maintenance
    g. Safety Procedures
  2. Care of Others
  3. Educational Activities
  4. Vocational Activities
    a. Vocational Exploration
    b. Job Acquisition
    c. Work or Job Performance
    d. Retirement Planning
    e. Volunteer Participation
C. Play or Leisure Activities
  1. Play or Leisure Exploration
  2. Play or Leisure Performance

II. Performance Components
A. Sensorimotor Component
  1. Sensory
    a. Sensory Awareness
    b. Sensory Processing
      (1) Tactile
      (2) Proprioceptive
      (3) Vestibular
      (4) Visual
      (5) Auditory
      (6) Gustatory
      (7) Olfactory
    c. Perceptual Processing
      (1) Stereognosis
      (2) Kinesthesia
      (3) Pain Response
      (4) Body Scheme
      (5) Right-Left Discrimination
      (6) Form Constancy
      (7) Position in Space
      (8) Visual-Closure
      (9) Figure Ground
     (10) Depth Perception
     (11) Spatial Relations
     (12) Topographical Orientation
  2. Neuromusculoskeletal
    a. Reflex
    b. Range of Motion
    c. Muscle Tone
    d. Strength
    e. Endurance

f. Postural Control
g. Postural Alignment
h. Soft Tissue Integrity
3. Motor
   a. Gross Coordination
   b. Crossing the Midline
   c. Laterality
   d. Bilateral Integration
   e. Motor Control
   f. Praxis
   g. Fine Motor Coordination/Dexterity
   h. Visual-Motor Integration
   i. Oral-Motor Control

B. Cognitive Integration and Cognitive Components
1. Level of Arousal
2. Orientation
3. Recognition
4. Attention Span
5. Initiation of Activity
6. Termination of Activity
7. Memory
8. Sequencing
9. Categorization
10. Concept Formation
11. Spatial Operations
12. Problem Solving
13. Learning
14. Generalization

C. Psychosocial Skills and Psychological Components
1. Psychological
   a. Values
   b. Interests
   c. Self-Concept
2. Social
   a. Role Performance
   b. Social Conduct
   c. Interpersonal skills
   d. Self-Expression
3. Self-Management
   a. Coping Skills
   b. Time Management
   c. Self-Control

III. Performance Contexts

A. Temporal Aspects
1. Chronological
2. Developmental
3. Life Cycle
4. Disability Status

B. Environment
1. Physical
2. Social
3. Cultural

Uniform Terminology for Occupational Therapy—Third Edition

"Occupational Therapy" is the use of purposeful activity or interventions to promote health and achieve functional outcomes. "Achieving functional outcomes" means to develop, improve, or restore the highest possible level of independence of any individual who is limited by a physical injury or illness, a dysfunctional condition, a cognitive impairment, a psychosocial dysfunction, a mental illness, a developmental or learning disability, or an adverse environmental condition. Assessment means the use of skilled observation or evaluation by the administration and interpretation of standardized or nonstandardized tests and measurements to identify areas for occupational therapy services.

Occupational therapy services include, but are not limited to:

1. the assessment, treatment, and education of or consultation with the individual, family, or other persons;
2. interventions directed toward developing, improving, or restoring daily living skills, work readiness or work performance, play skills or leisure capacities, or enhancing educational performances skills; or
3. providing for the development, improvement, or restoration of sensorimotor, oral-motor, perceptual or neuromuscular functioning; or emotional, motivational, cognitive, or psychosocial components of performance.

These services may require assessment of the need for and use of interventions such as the design, development, adaptation, application, or training in the use of assistive technology devices; the design, fabrication, or application of rehabilitative technology such as selected orthotic devices; training in the use of assistive technology, orthotic or prosthetic devices; the application of physical agent modalities as an adjunct to or in preparation for purposeful activity; the use of ergonomic principles; the adaptation of environments and processes to enhance functional performance; or the promotion of health and wellness (AOTA, 1993, p. 1117).

I. Performance Areas

Throughout this document, activities have been described as if individuals performed the tasks themselves. Occupational therapy also recognizes that individuals arrange for tasks to be done through others. The profession views independence as the ability to self-determine activity performance, regardless of who actually performs the activity.

A. *Activities of Daily Living*—Self-maintenance tasks.
1. *Grooming*—Obtaining and using supplies; removing body hair (use of razors, tweezers, lotions, etc.); applying and removing cosmetics; washing, drying, combing, styling, and brushing hair; caring for nails (hands and feet), caring for skin, ears, and eyes; and applying deodorant.
2. *Oral Hygiene*—Obtaining and using supplies; cleaning mouth; brushing and flossing teeth; or removing, cleaning and reinserting dental orthotics and prosthetics.
3. *Bathing/Showering*—Obtaining and using supplies; soaping, rinsing, and drying all body parts; maintaining bathing position; transferring to and from bathing positions.
4. *Toilet Hygiene*—Obtaining and using supplies; clothing management; maintaining toileting position; transferring to and from toileting position; cleaning body; and caring for menstrual and continence needs (including catheters, colostomies, and suppository management).
5. *Personal Device Care*—Cleaning and maintaining personal care items, such as

172

hearing aids, contact lenses, glasses, orthotics, prosthetics, adaptive equipment, and contraceptive and sexual devices.

6. *Dressing*—Selecting clothing and accessories appropriate for the time of day, weather, and occasion; obtaining clothing from storage area; dressing and undressing in a sequential fashion; fastening and adjusting clothing and shoes; and applying and removing personal devices, prostheses, or orthoses.

7. *Feeding and Eating*—Setting up food; selecting and using appropriate utensils and tableware; bringing food or drink to mouth; sucking, masticating, coughing, and swallowing; and management of alternative methods or nourishment.

8. *Medication Routine*—Obtaining medication, opening and closing containers, following prescribed schedules, taking correct quantities, reporting problems and adverse effects, and administering correct quantities using prescribed methods.

9. *Health Maintenance*—Developing and maintaining routines for illness prevention and wellness promotion, such as physical fitness, nutrition, and decreasing health risk behaviors.

10. *Socialization*—Accessing opportunities and interacting with other people in appropriate contextual and cultural ways to meet emotional and physical needs.

11. *Functional Communication*—Using equipment or systems to send and receive information, such as writing equipment, telephones, typewriters, communication boards, call lights, emergency systems, Braille writers, telecommunication devices for the deaf, and augmentative communication systems.

12. *Functional Mobility*—Moving from one position or place to another, such as in-bed mobility, wheelchair mobility, transfers (wheelchair, bed, car, tub/shower, toilet, chair, floor); performing functional ambulation and transporting objects.

13. *Community Mobility*—Moving self in the community and using public or private transportation, such as driving, or accessing buses, taxi cabs, or other public transportation systems.

14. *Emergency Response*—Recognizing sudden, unexpected hazardous situations, and initiating action to reduce the threat to health and safety.

15. *Sexual Expression*—Engaging in desired sexual activities.

B. *Work and Productive Activities*—Purposeful activities for self-development, social contribution, and livelihood.

1. *Home Management*—Obtaining and maintaining personal and household possessions and environment.

   a. *Clothing Care*—Obtaining and using supplies; sorting, laundering (hand, machine, and dry clean); folding; ironing; storing; and mending.

   b. *Cleaning*—Obtaining and using supplies; picking up; putting away; vacuuming; sweeping and mopping floors; dusting; polishing; scrubbing; washing windows; cleaning mirrors; making beds; and removing trash and recyclables.

   c. *Meal Preparation and Cleanup*—Planning nutritious meals; preparing and serving food; opening and closing containers, cabinets, and drawers; using kitchen utensils and appliances; cleaning up and storing food safely.

   d. *Shopping*—Preparing shopping lists (grocery and other); selecting and purchasing items; selecting method of payment; and completing money transactions.

   e. *Money Management*—Budgeting, paying bills, and using bank systems.

   f. *Household Maintenance*—Maintaining home, yard, garden appliances, vehicles, and household items.

   g. *Safety Procedures*—Knowing and performing preventive and emergency procedures to maintain a safe environment and prevent injuries.

2. *Care of Others*—Providing for children, spouse, parents, pets or others, such as the physical care, nurturing, communicating, and using age-appropriate activities.

3. *Educational Activities*—Participating in a learning environment through school, community, or work-sponsored activities, such as exploring educational interests,

attending to instruction, managing assignments, and contributing to group experiences.

4. *Vocational Activities*—Participating in work-related activities.

a. *Vocational Exploration*—Determining aptitudes, developing interests and skills, and selecting appropriate vocational pursuits.

b. *Job Acquisition*—Identifying and selecting work opportunities, and completing application and interview processes.

c. *Work or Job Performance*—Performing job tasks in a timely and effective manner; incorporating necessary work behaviors.

d. *Retirement Planning*—Determining aptitudes, developing interests and skills, and identifying appropriate avocational pursuits.

e. *Volunteer Participation*—Performing unpaid activities for the benefit of selected individuals, groups, or causes.

C. *Play or Leisure Activities*—Intrinsically motivating activities for amusement, relaxation, spontaneous enjoyment, or self-expression.

1. *Play or Leisure Exploration*—Identifying interests, skills, opportunities, and appropriate play or leisure activities.

2. *Play or Leisure Performance*—Planning and participating in play or leisure activities; maintaining a balance of play or leisure activities with work and productive activities, and activities of daily living; obtaining, utilizing, and maintaining equipment and supplies.

II. Performance Components

A. *Sensorimotor Component*—The ability to receive input, process information, and produce output.

1. *Sensory*

a. *Sensory Awareness*—Receiving and differentiating sensory stimuli.

b. *Sensory Processing*—Interpreting sensory stimuli.

(1) *Tactile*—Interpreting light touch, pressure, temperature, pain, and vibration through skin contact/receptors.

(2) *Proprioceptive*—Interpreting stimuli originating in muscles, joints, and other internal tissues to give information about the position of one body part in relation to another.

(3) *Vestibular*—Interpreting stimuli from the inner ear receptors regarding head position and movement.

(4) *Visual*—Interpreting stimuli through the eyes, including peripheral vision and acuity, awareness of color and pattern.

(5) *Auditory*—Interpreting and localizing sounds, and discriminating background sounds.

(6) *Gustatory*—Interpreting tastes.

(7) *Olfactory*—Interpreting odors.

c. *Perceptual Processing*—Organizing sensory input into meaningful patterns.

(1) *Stereognosis*—Identifying objects through proprioception, cognition, and the sense of touch.

(2) *Kinesthesia*—Identifying the excursion and direction of joint movement.

(3) *Pain Response*—Interpreting noxious stimuli.

(4) *Body Scheme*—Acquiring an internal awareness of the body and the relationship of body parts to each other.

(5) *Right-Left Discrimination*—Differentiating one side of the body from the other.

(6) *Form Constancy*—Recognizing forms and objects as the same in various environments, positions, and sizes.

(7) *Position in Space*—Determining the spatial relationship of figures and objects to self or other forms and objects.

(8) *Visual-Closure*—Identifying forms or objects from incomplete presentations.

(9) *Figure Ground*—Differentiating between foreground and background forms and objects.

(10) *Depth Perception*—Determining the relative distance between objects, figures, or landmarks and the observer, and changes in planes of surfaces.

(11) *Spatial Relations*—Determining the position of objects relative to each other.

(12) *Topographical Orientation*—Determining the location of objects and settings and the route to the location.

2. *Neuromusculoskeletal*

   a. *Reflex*—Eliciting an involuntary muscle response by sensory input.

   b. *Range of Motion*—Moving body parts through an arc.

   c. *Muscle Tone*—Demonstrating a degree of tension or resistance in a muscle at rest and in response to stretch.

   d. *Strength*—Demonstrating a degree of muscle power when movement is resisted, as with objects or gravity.

   e. *Endurance*—Sustaining cardiac, pulmonary, and musculoskeletal exertion over time.

   f. *Postural Control*—Using righting and equilibrium adjustments to maintain balance during functional movements.

   g. *Postural Alignment*—Maintaining biomechanical integrity among body parts.

   h. *Soft Tissue Integrity*—Maintaining anatomical and physiological condition of interstitial tissue and skin.

3. *Motor*

   a. *Gross Coordination*—Using large muscle groups for controlled, goal-directed movements.

   b. *Crossing the Midline*—Moving limbs and eyes across the midsagittal plane of the body.

   c. *Laterality*—Using a preferred unilateral body part for activities requiring a high level of skill.

   d. *Bilateral Integration*—Coordinating both body sides during activity.

   e. *Motor Control*—Using the body in functional and versatile movement patterns.

   f. *Praxis*—Conceiving and planning a new motor act in response to an environmental demand.

   g. *Fine Coordination/Dexterity*—Using small muscle groups for controlled movements, particularly in object manipulation.

   h. *Visual-Motor Integration*—Coordinating the interaction of information from the eyes with body movement during activity.

   i. *Oral-Motor Control*—Coordinating oropharyngeal musculature for controlled movements.

B. *Cognitive Integration and Cognitive Components*

1. *Level of Arousal*—Demonstrating alertness and responsiveness to environmental stimuli.

2. *Orientation*—Identifying person, place, time, and situation.

3. *Recognition*—Identifying familiar faces, objects, and other previously presented materials.

4. *Attention Span*—Focusing on a task over time.

5. *Initiation of Activity*—Starting a physical or mental activity.

6. *Termination of Activity*—Stopping an activity at an appropriate time.

7. *Memory*—Recalling information after brief or long periods of time.

8. *Sequencing*—Placing information, concepts, and actions in order.

9. *Categorization*—Identifying similarities of and differences among pieces of environmental information.

10. *Concept Formation*—Organizing a variety of information to form thoughts and

ideas.

11. *Spatial Operations*—Mentally manipulating the position of objects in various relationships.
12. *Problem Solving*—Recognizing a problem, defining a problem, identifying alternative plans, selecting a plan, organizing steps in a plan, implementing a plan, and evaluating the outcome.
13. *Learning*—Acquiring new concepts and behaviors.
14. *Generalization*—Applying previously learned concepts and behaviors to a variety of new situations.

C. *Psychosocial Skills and Psychological Components*—The ability to interact in society and to process emotions.

1. *Psychological*
   a. *Values*—Identifying ideas or beliefs that are important to self and others.
   b. *Interests*—Identifying mental or physical activities that create pleasure and maintain attention.
   c. *Self-Concept*—Developing the value of the physical, emotional, and sexual self.

2. *Social*
   a. *Role Performance*—Identifying, maintaining, and balancing functions one assumes or acquires in society (e.g., worker, student, parent, friend, religious participant).
   b. *Social Conduct*—Interacting using manners, personal space, eye contact, gestures, active listening, and self-expression appropriate to one's environment.
   c. *Interpersonal Skills*—Using verbal and nonverbal communication to interact in a variety of settings.
   d. *Self-Expression*—Using a variety of styles and skills to express thoughts, feelings, and needs.

3. *Self-Management*
   a. *Coping Skills*—Identifying and managing stress and related reactors.
   b. *Time Management*—Planning and participating in a balance of self-care, work, leisure, and rest activities to promote satisfaction and health.
   c. *Self-Control*—Modifying one's own behavior in response to environmental needs, demands, constraints, personal aspirations, and feedback from others.

III. Performance Contexts

Assessment of function in performance areas is greatly influenced by the contexts in which the individual must perform. Occupational therapy practitioners consider performance contexts when determining feasibility and appropriateness of interventions. Occupational therapy practitioners may choose interventions based on an understanding of contexts, or may choose interventions directly aimed at altering the contexts to improve performance.

A. *Temporal Aspects*
   1. *Chronological*—Individual's age.
   2. *Developmental*—Stage or phase of maturation.
   3. *Life Cycle*—Place in important life phases, such as career cycle, parenting cycle, or educational process.
   4. *Disability Status*—Place in continuum of disability, such as acuteness of injury, chronicity of disability, or terminal nature of illness.

B. *Environment*
   1. *Physical*—Nonhuman aspects of contexts. Includes the accessibility to and performance within environments having natural terrain, plants, animals, buildings, furniture, objects, tools, or devices.
   2. *Social*—Availability and expectations of significant individuals, such as spouse, friends, and caregivers. Also includes larger social groups which are influential in establishing norms, role expectations, and social routines.

3. *Cultural*—Customs, beliefs, activity patterns, behavior standards, and expectations accepted by the society of which the individual is a member. Includes political aspects, such as laws that affect access to resources and affirm personal rights. Also includes opportunities for education, employment, and economic support.

References

American Occupational Therapy Association. (1979). *Occupational therapy output reporting system and uniform terminology for reporting occupational therapy services.* Rockville, MD: Author.

American Occupational Therapy Association. (1989). Uniform terminology for occupational therapy—Second edition. *American Journal of Occupational Therapy, 43,* 808-815.

American Occupational Therapy Association. (1993). Definition of occupational therapy practice for state regulation (Policy 5.3.1). *American Journal of Occupational Therapy, 47,* 1117-1121.

Authors:

The Terminology Task Force:

Winifred Dunn, PhD, OTR, FAOTA—Chairperson

Mary Foto, OTR, FAOTA

Jim Hinojosa, PhD, OTR, FAOTA

Barbara Schell, PhD, OTR/L, FAOTA

Linda Kohlman Thomson, MOT, OTR, OT(C), FAOTA

Sarah D. Hertfelder, MEd, MOT, OTR/L—Staff Liaison

for The Commission on Practice

Jim Hinojosa, PhD, OTR, FAOTA—Chairperson

Adopted by the Representative Assembly 7/94

NOTE: This document replaces the following documents, all of which were rescinded by the 1994 Representative Assembly:

Occupational Therapy Product Output Reporting System (1979)
Uniform Terminology for Reporting Occupational Therapy Services—First Edition (1979)
Uniform Occupational Therapy Evaluation Checklist (1981)
Uniform Terminology for Occupational Therapy—Second Edition (1989)

Uniform Terminology—Third Edition: Application to Practice

Introduction

This document was developed to help occupational therapists apply *Uniform Terminology, Third Edition* to practice. The original grid format (Dunn, 1988) enabled occupational therapy practitioners to systematically identify deficit and strength areas of an individual and to select appropriate activities to address these areas in occupational therapy intervention (Dunn & McGourty, 1990). For the third edition, the profession is highlighting "Contexts" as another critical aspect of performance. A second grid provides therapy practitioners with a mechanism to consider the contextual features of performance in practitioners with a mechanism to consider the contextual features of performance in activities of daily living (ADL), work and productive activity, and play/leisure. "Performance Areas" and "Performance Components" (Figure A) focus on the individual. These features are embedded in the "Performance Contexts" (Figure B).

On the original grid (Dunn, 1988), the horizontal axis contains the Performance Areas of Activities of Daily Living, Work and Productive Activities, and Play or Leisure Activities (see Figure A). These Performance Areas are the functional outcomes occupational therapy addresses. The vertical axis contains the Performance Components, including Sensorimotor Components, Cognitive Components, and Psychosocial Components. The Performance Components are the skills and abilities that an individual uses to engage in the Performance Areas. During an occupational therapy assessment, the occupational therapy practitioner determines an individual's abilities and limitations in the Performance Components and how they affect the individual's functional outcomes in the Performance Areas.

Figure A—Uniform Terminology Grid
(Performance Areas and Performance Components)
Performance Areas

I. Performance Components
    A. Sensorimotor Component
        1. Sensory
            a. Sensory Awareness
            b. Sensory Processing
                (1) Tactile
                (2) Proprioceptive
                (3) Vestibular
                (4) Visual
                (5) Auditory
                (6) Gustatory
                (7) Olfactory
            c. Perceptual Processing
                (1) Stereognosis
                (2) Kinesthesia
                (3) Pain Response
                (4) Body Scheme
                (5) Right-Left Discrimination
                (6) Form Constancy
                (7) Position in Space
                (8) Visual-Closure
                (9) Figure Ground
                (10) Depth Perception
                (11) Spatial Relations
                (12) Topographical Orientation
        2. Neuromusculoskeletal
            a. Reflex
            b. Range of Motion
            c. Muscle Tone

    d. Strength
    e. Endurance
    f. Postural Control
    g. Postural Alignment
    h. Soft Tissue Integrity
  3. Motor
    a. Gross Coordination
    b. Crossing the Midline
    c. Laterality
    d. Bilateral Integration
    e. Motor Control
    f. Praxis
    g. Fine Coordination/Dexterity
    h. Visual-Motor Integration
    i. Oral-Motor Control
B. Cognitive Integration and Cognitive Components
  1. Level of Arousal
  2. Orientation
  3. Recognition
  4. Attention Span
  5. Initiation of Activity
  6. Termination of Activity
  7. Memory
  8. Sequencing
  9. Categorization
  10. Concept Formation
  11. Spatial Operations
  12. Problem Solving
  13. Learning
  14. Generalization
C. Psychosocial Skills and Psychological Components
  1. Psychological
    a. Values
    b. Interests
    c. Self-Concept
  2. Social
    a. Role Performance
    b. Social Conduct
    c. Interpersonal Skills
    d. Self-Expression
  3. Self-Management
    a. Coping Skills
    b. Time Management
    c. Self-Control

SPECIAL NOTE: The first application document (Dunn & McGourty, 1989) describes how to use the original *Uniform Terminology* grid with a variety of individuals. It is quite useful to introduce these concepts. However, the third edition of *Uniform Terminology* contains some changes in the Performance Areas and Performance Components lists. Be sure to check for the terminology currently approved in the third edition before applying this information in current practice environments.

With the addition of Performance Contexts into *Uniform Terminology*, occupational therapy practitioners must consider how to interface what the individual wants to do (i.e.,

Figure B illustrates the interaction of Performance Areas and Performance Contexts as a model for therapists' planning.

Figure B—Uniform Terminology Grid
(Performance Areas and Performance Contexts)
Performance Areas

I. Performance Contexts
    A. Temporal Aspects
        1. Chronological
        2. Developmental
        3. Life Cycle
        4. Disability Status
    B. Environment
        1. Physical
        2. Social
        3. Cultural

The grid in Figure B can be used to analyze the contexts of performance for a particular individual. For example, when working with a toddler with a developmental disability who needs to learn to eat, the occupational therapy practitioner would consider all the Performance Contexts features as they might impact on this toddler's ability to master eating. Unlike the grid in Figure A, in which the occupational therapy practitioner selects *both* Performance Areas (i.e., what the individual wants or needs to do) and the Performance Component (i.e., a person's strengths and needs), in this grid (Figure B) the occupational therapy practitioner only selects the Performance Area. After the Performance Area is identified through collaboration with the individual and significant others, the occupational therapy practitioner considers ALL Performance Context features as they might impact on performance of the selected task.

Intervention Planning

Intervention planning occurs both within the general domain of concern of occupational therapy (i.e., uniform terminology) and by considering the profession's theoretical frames of reference that offer insights about how to approach the problem. In Figure A, the occupational therapy practitioner considers the Performance Areas that are of interest to the individual and the individual's strengths and concerns within the Performance Components. The intervention strategies would emerge from the cells on the grid that are placed at the intersection of the Performance Areas and the targeted Performance Components (strength and/or concern). For example, if a child needed to improve sensory processing and fine coordination for oral hygiene and grooming, an occupational therapy practitioner might select a sensory integrative frame of reference to create intervention strategies, such as adding textures to handles and teaching the child sand and bean digging games. Dunn and McGourty (1989) discuss this in more detail.

When using Figure B, the occupational therapy practitioner considers the Performance Contexts features in relation to the desired Performance Area. The occupational therapy practitioner would analyze the individual's temporal, physical, social, and cultural contexts to determine the relevance of particular interventions. For example, if the child mentioned above was a member of a family in which having messy hands from sand play was unacceptable, the occupational therapy practitioner would consider alternate strategies that are more compatible with their lifestyle. For example, perhaps the family would be more interested in developing puppet play. This would still provide the child with opportunities to experience the textures of various puppets and the hand movements required to manipulate the puppets in play context, without adding the messiness of sand. When occupational therapy practitioners consider contexts, interventions become more relevant and applicable to individual's lives.

Case Example 1

Sophie, a 75-year-old lady who was widowed 3 years ago, is recovering from a cerebral vascular accident and has been transferred from an acute care unit to an inpatient medical rehabilitation unit. Prior to her admission, she was living in a small house in an isolated location and has no family living nearby. She was driving independently and frequently ran errands for her friends. She is adamant in her goal to return to her home after discharge. All of her friends are quite elderly and are not able to provide many resources for support.

Sophie and the team collaborated to identify her goals. Sophie decided that she wanted to be able to meet her daily needs with little or no assistance. Almost all of the Performance Areas are critical in order to achieve the outcome of community living in her own home. Being able to cook all of her meals, bathe independently, and have alternative transportation available is necessary. Because of their significant impact on the patient's function in the Performance Areas, some of the Performance Components that may need to be addressed are figure ground, muscle tone, postural control, fine coordination, memory, and self-management.

In the selection of occupational therapy interventions, it is critical to analyze the elements of Performance Contexts for the individual. The physical and social elements of her home environment do not support returning home without modifications to her home and additional social supports being established. Railings must be added to the front steps, provision of and instruction in the use of a tub seat, and instruction in the use of specialized transportation may need to occur. If this same individual had been living in an apartment in a retirement community prior to her CVA, the contexts of performance would support a return home with fewer environmental modifications being needed. Being independent in cooking might not be necessary due to meals being provided, and the bathroom might already be accessible and safe. If the individual had friends and family available, the social support network might already be established to assist with shopping and transportation needs. The occupational therapy interventions would be different due to the contexts in which the individual will be performing. Interventions must be selected with the impact of the Performance Contexts as an essential element.

Case Example 2

Malcolm is a 9-year-old boy who has a learning disability which causes him to have a variety of problems in school. His teachers complain that he is difficult to manage in the classroom. Some of the Performance Components that may need to be addressed are his self-control such as interrupting, difficulty sitting during instruction, and difficulty with peer relations. Other children avoid him on the playground, because he doesn't follow rules, doesn't play fair, and tends to anger quickly when confronted. The performance component impairment with concept formation is reflected in his sloppy and disorganized classroom assignments.

The critical elements of the Performance Contexts are the temporal aspect of age-appropriateness of his behavior and the social environment aspect of his immature socialization. The significant cultural and temporal aspects of his family are that they place a high premium on athletic prowess.

The occupational therapy practitioner intervenes in several ways to address his behavior in the school environment. The occupational therapy practitioner focuses on structuring the classroom environment and facilitating consistent behavioral expectations structuring the classroom environment and facilitating consistent behavioral expectations for Malcolm by educational personnel. She also consults with the teachers to develop ways to structure activities which will support his ability to relate to other children in a positive way.

In contrast, another child with similar learning disabilities, but who is 12 years old and in the 7th grade might have different concerns. Elements of the Performance Contexts are the temporal aspect of the age-appropriateness of his behavior; and the social environment context of school where "bullying" behavior is unacceptable and in which completing assignments is expected. In addressing the cultural Performance Contexts the occupational therapy practitioner recognizes from meeting the parents that they have only average expectation for academic performance but value athletic accomplishments.

Since teachers at his school consider completion of home assignments to be part of average performance, the occupational therapy practitioner works with the child and parents on time management and reinforcement strategies to meet this expectation. After consultation with the coach, she works with the father to create activities to improve his athletic abilities. When occupational therapy practitioners consider family values as part of the contexts of performance, different intervention priorities may emerge.

Authors:

The Terminology Task Force:

Winnie Dunn, PhD, OTR, FAOTA—Chairperson

Mary Foto, OTR, FAOTA

Jim Hinojosa, PhD, OTR, FAOTA

Barbara A. Boyt Schell, PhD, OTR/L, FAOTA

Linda Kohlman Thomson, MOT, OTR, OT(C), FAOTA

Sarah D. Hertfelder, MEd, MOT, OTR/L—Staff Liaison

for The Commission on Practice—1994

Jim Hinojosa, PhD, OTR, FAOTA—Chairperson

NOTE: This document replaces the 1989 *Application of Uniform Terminology to Practice* that accompanied the *Uniform Terminology for Occupational Therapy—Second Edition*.

Appendix E

STUDENT WORKSHEETS

Form 2-1.
ACTIVITY AWARENESS FORM

Student: _____ Date: _____

Activity: _____

Course: _____

Directions: Reflecting on the activity just performed, complete the following sentences with the first thoughts that come to mind.

1. During this activity I was thinking about. . .

2. While doing this activity I felt like. . .

3. In doing this activity, the parts of my body I remember using were. . .

4. To do this activity I need to. . .(mentally, emotionally, physically)

5. When I do this activity again I will. . .

6. From doing this activity I became aware of. . .

Form 2-3.
ACTION IDENTIFICATION FORM

Directions: Select an activity and list the major actions (in sequence) required for you to perform this activity *in ten or less steps* . Repeat the exercise after observing someone else perform the same activity. Use the "Do-What-How" format.

Student: _____ Date: _____

Activity selected: _____

Course: _____

Observation of Self	Observation of Another

Form 2-5.
ACTIVITY ANALYSIS FORM

Student: _____ Date: _____

Course: _____

Part I - Activity Summary
Directions: Respond to the following in list format.

1. Name of activity

2. Brief description of activity

3. Tools/equipment (non-expendable), cost, and source

4. Materials/supplies (expendable), cost and source

5. Space/environmental requirements

6. Sequence of major steps; time required to complete each step

7. Precautions (review "Sequence of major steps")

8. Contraindications (review participant's status)

9. Special considerations (age appropriateness, educational requirements, cultural relevance, sexual identification, other)

10. Acceptable criteria for completed project

Part II - Occupational Performance Components
Directions: Indicate the skill components necessary to complete the task (as it is normally done). State your reasoning to the right of each item. Write "N/A" if not applicable. Refer to Uniform Terminology (Appendix B) for definitions of terms.

A. Sensorimotor Components
    1. Neuromuscular
        a. Reflex integration

        b. Range of motion
            (1) active

            (2) passive

            (3) active assistive

        c. Gross and fine coordination
            (1) muscle control

            (2) coordination

            (3) dexterity

        d. Strength and endurance
            (1) building strength, cardiopulmonary reserve

            (2) increasing length of work period

            (3) decreasing fatigue/strain

    2. Sensory integration
        a. Sensory awareness
            (1) tactile awareness

            (2) stereognosis

            (3) kinesthesia

            (4) proprioceptive awareness

            (5) ocular control

            (6) vestibular awareness

            (7) auditory awareness

            (8) gustatory awareness

            (9) olfactory awareness

Form 2-5. (continued)

   b. Visual-spatial awareness
     (1) figure-ground

     (2) form constancy

     (3) position in space

   c. Body integration
     (1) body schema

     (2) postural balance

     (3) bilateral motor coordination

     (4) right-left discrimination

     (5) visual-motor integration

     (6) crossing the midline

     (7) praxis

B. Cognitive Components
  1. Orientation

  2. Conceptualization/comprehension
   a. Concentration

   b. Attention span

   c. Memory

  3. Cognitive integration
   a. Generalization

   b. Problem solving
     (1) defining or evaluating the problem

     (2) organizing a plan

     (3) making decisions/judgment

     (4) implementing a plan

     (5) evaluating decision/judgment

C. Psychosocial Components
   1. Self-management
      a. Self-expression
         (1) experiencing/recognizing a range of emotions

         (2) having an adequate vocabulary

         (3) writing and speaking skills

         (4) use of nonverbal signs and symbols

      b. Self-control
         (1) observing own and others' behavior

         (2) recognizing need for behavior/action change

         (3) imitating new behaviors

         (4) directing energies into stress-reducing behaviors

   2. Dyadic interaction
      a. Understanding norms of communication and interaction

      b. Setting limits on self and others

      c. Compromising and negotiating

      d. Handling stress

      e. Cooperating and competing with others

      f. Responsibly relying on self and others

Form 2-5. (continued)

   3. Group interaction
      a. Performing social/emotional roles and tasks

      b. Understanding simple group process

      c. Participating in a mutually beneficial group

D. Task Requirements
   1. Work patterns
      a. Light

      b. Moderate

      c. Heavy

   2. Method
      a. Structured

      b. Methodical

      c. Repetitive

      d. Expressive

      e. Creative

      f. Orderly

      g. Physical contact

      h. Projective

Part III - Occupational Performance
Directions: Indicate possible treatment goals that this activity might address in one or more of the areas of occupational performance. State your reasoning as in Part I. Write "N/A" if not applicable.

A. Independent Living/Daily Living Skills
  1. Physical daily living skills
     a. Grooming and hygiene

     b. Feeding/eating

     c. Dressing

     d. Functional mobility

     e. Functional communication

     f. Object manipulation

  2. Psychological/emotional daily living skills
     a. Self-concept/self-identity

     b. Situational coping

     c. Community involvement

  3. Work
     a. Homemaking

     b. Child care/parenting

     c. Employment preparation

  4. Play/leisure
     a. Recognizing one's needs

     b. Identifying characteristics of play

     c. Selecting play activities

     d. Adaptation of activities

     e. Utilizing community resources

Part IV - Occupational Performance Modifications
Directions: Indicate ways this activity might be modified to increase independent function.
State your reasoning. Write "N/A" if not applicable.

Note: This activity should be done with the non-dominant hand only.

A. Therapeutic Adaptations
    1. Orthotics
        a. Static or dynamic positioning

        b. Relief of pain

        c. Maintain joint alignment

        d. Protect joint integrity

        e. Improve function

        f. Decrease deformity

    2. Prosthetics

    3. Assistive/adaptive equipment
        a. Architectural modification

        b. Environmental modification

        c. Assistive equipment

        d. Wheelchair modification

B. Prevention
    1. Energy conservation
        a. Energy-saving procedures

        b. Activity restriction

        c. Work simplification

        d. Time management

        e. Environmental organization

2. Joint protection/body mechanics
   a. Proper body mechanics

   b. Avoiding static/deforming postures

   c. Avoiding excessive weight bearing

   d. Positioning

   e. Coordinating daily living activities

Implications for Treatment

Directions: Explain how and for whom this activity could be beneficial. Indicate physical and/or psychosocial dysfunction.

Grading the Activity

Directions: Describe ways you might grade this activity in terms of:

1. Duration/endurance

2. Range of motion

3. Resistance

4. Complexity

5. Independence

Form 2-7.
PATIENT-ACTIVITY CORRELATION FORM

Student: _____

Course: _____ Date: _____

1. Patient Profile

2. Therapeutic Goals
    a. Long Term

    b. Short Term

3. Goal-Directed Activity Description

4. Activity Preparation Requirements
    a. Task

    b. Personnel

    c. Preparation time

    d. Place/space

    e. Materials

    f. Equipment

    g. Safety precautions (personnel)

5. Activity Implementation Requirements
   a. Personnel

   b. Setting/location

   c. Area/space

   d. Environment

   e. Materials

   f. Equipment/adaptations

   g. Time frame

   h. Safety precautions (patient)

6. Activity Sequence (Action steps: ten or less)

7. Therapeutic Applications (UTS)

Form 4-1.
APPLICATION OF PATIENT-ACTIVITY CORRELATION TO A CASE STUDY

1. Patient Profile

   a. Personal data:
      (1) Age _____ Sex_____ Marital Status _____
      (2) Occupation: _____
      (3) Diagnosis: _____

   b. Medical history (etiology, prognosis, symptomatology, medical and ancillary treatment)

   c. Screening/evaluation procedures

2. Therapeutic Goals: Long- and Short-term

3. Treatment Modalities

4. Progress

5. Discharge Summary

6. Following the presentation the student will determine Uniform Terminology
   a. Occupational performance area(s)

   b. Occupational performance components

7. Roles
   a. OTR

   b. COTA

Appendix F

SUGGESTED JOURNAL READINGS

Adelstein, L.A. & Nelson, D.L. (1985). Effects of sharing versus non-sharing on affective meaning in collage activities. *Occupational Therapy in Mental Health, 5,* 29-45.

Allen, C. (1982). Independence through activity: The practice of occupational therapy (psychiatry). *American Journal of Occupational Therapy, 36,* 731-739.

Banning, M.R. & Nelson, D.L. (1987). The effects of activity-elicited humor and group structure on group cohesion and affective meanings. *American Journal of Occupational Therapy, 41,* 510-514.

Bissell, J. & Mailloux, Z. (1981). The use of crafts in occupational therapy for the physically disabled. *American Journal of Occupational Therapy, 35,* 369-374.

Carter, B.A., Nelson, D.L. & Duncombe, L.W. (1983). The effect of psychological type on the mood and meaning of two collage activities. *American Journal of Occupational Therapy, 39,* 688-693.

Chandani, A. & Hill, C. (1990). What really is therapeutic activity? *The British Journal of Occupational Therapy, 53,* 15-18.

Clark, P.N. (1979). Human development through occupation: Theoretical frameworks in contemporary occupational therapy practice. *American Journal of Occupational Therapy, 33,* 505-514.

DiJoseph, L. (1982). Independence through activity: Mind, body, and environment interaction in therapy. *American Journal of Occupational Therapy, 36,* 740-744.

Dunn, W. (1982). Independence through activity: The practice of occupational therapy (pediatrics). *American Journal of Occupational Therapy, 36* 745-747.

Dunn, W. & McGourty, L. (1989). Application of uniform terminology to practice. *The American Journal of Occupational Therapy, 43,* 817-831.

Dunton, W.R. Jr. (1923). A debate upon toy-making as a therapeutic occupation: Con. *Archives of Occupational Therapy, 2,* 39-43.

Dunton, W.R. Jr. (1923). Rejoiner. *Archives of Occupational Therapy, 2,* 47.

Fahl, M.A. (1970). Emotionally disturbed children: Effects of cooperative and competitive activity on peer interaction. *American Journal of Occupational Therapy, 24,* 31-33.

Fidler, G.S. (1948). Psychological evaluation of occupational therapy activities. *American Journal of Occupational Therapy, 2,* 284-287.

Fidler, G.S. (1969). The Task-oriented group as a context for treatment. *American Journal of Occupational Therapy, 23,* 43-48.

Fidler, G.S. (1981). From crafts to competence. *American Journal of Occupational Therapy, 35,* 567-573.

Fitts, H.A. & Howe, M.C. (1987). Use of leisure time by cardiac patients. *American Journal of Occupational Therapy, 41,* 583-589.

Fox, J. & Jirgal, D. (1967). Therapeutic properties of activities as examined by the clinical council of the Wisconsin schools of O.T. *American Journal of Occupational Therapy, 21,* 29-33.

Froehlich, J. & Nelson, D.L. (1986). Affective meanings of life review through activities and discussion. *American Journal of Occupational Therapy, 40,* 27-33.

Hatter, J.K. & Nelson, D.L. (1987). Altruism and task participation in the elderly. *American Journal of Occupational Therapy, 41,* 379-381.

Henry, A.D., Nelson, D.L. & Duncombe, L.W. (1984). Choice-making in group and individual activity. *American Journal of Occupational Therapy, 38,* 245-251.

Huss, J. (1981). From kinesiology to adaptation. *American Journal of Occupational Therapy, 35,* 574-580.

Kielhofner, G. & Burke, J.P. (1980). A model of human occupation, Part 1. Conceptual framework and content. *American Journal of Occupational Therapy, 34,* 572-581.

Kielhofner, G. (1980). A model of human occupation, Part 2. Ontogenesis perspective of temporal adaptation. *American Journal of Occupational Therapy, 34,* 657-663.

Kielhofner, G. (1980). A model of human occupation, Part 3. Benign and vicious cycles. *American Journal of Occupational Therapy, 34,* 731-737.

Kielhofner, G., Burke, J.P. & Igi, C.H. (1980). A model of human occupation, Part 4. Assessment and intervention. *American Journal of Occupational Therapy, 34,* 777-788.

Kielhofner, G. (1982). A heritage of activity: Development of theory. *American Journal of Occupational Therapy, 36,* 723-730.

Kircher, M.A. (1984). Motivation as a factor of perceived exertion in purposeful versus nonpurposeful activity. *American Journal of Occupational Therapy, 38,* 165-170.

Kleinman, B.L. & Stalcup, A. (1991). The effect of a graded craft activities on visuomotor integration in an inpatient child psychiatry population. *American Journal of Occupational Therapy, 45,* 324-330.

Kremer, E.R.H., Nelson, D.L. & Duncombe, L.W. (1984). Effects of selected activities on affective meaning in psychiatric clients. *American Journal of Occupational Therapy, 38,* 522-528.

Licht, S. (1947). Kinetic analysis of crafts and occupations. *Occupational Therapy and Rehabilitation, 26,* 75-78.

Llorens, L.A. (1973). Activity analysis for cognitive-perceptual motor dysfunction. *American Journal of Occupational Therapy, 27,* 453-456.

Llorens, L.A. (1986). Activity analysis: Agreement among factors in a sensory processing model. *American Journal of Occupational Therapy, 40,* 103-110.

Lyons, B.G. (1983). Purposeful versus human activity. *American Journal of Occupational Therapy, 37,* 493-495.

Meyer, A. (1922). Philosophy of occupational therapy. *Archives of Occupational Therapy, 1,* 1-10.

Miller, L. & Nelson, D.L. (1987). Dual-purpose activity versus single-purpose activity in terms of duration on task, exertion level, and affect. *Occupational Therapy in Mental Health, 7,* 55-67.

Mullins, C.S., Nelson, D.L. & Smith, D.A. (1987). Exercise through dual-purpose activity in the institutionalized elderly. *Physical and Occupational Therapy in Geriatrics, 5,* 29-39.

Mumford, M. (1974). A Comparison of interpersonal skills in verbal and activity groups. *American Journal of Occupational Therapy, 28,* 281-283.

Nelson, D.L. (1988). Occupation: Form and performance. *The American Journal of Occupational Therapy, 42,* 633-641.

Nelson, D.L., Peterson, C., Smith, D.A., Boughton, J.A. & Whalen, G.M. (1988). Effects of project versus parallel groups on social interaction and affective responses in senior citizens. *American Journal of Occupational Therapy, 42,* 23-29.

Nelson, D.L., Thompson, G. & Moore, J.A. (1982). Identification of factors of affective meaning in four selected activities. *American Journal of Occupational Therapy, 36,* 381-387.

Niswander, P. & Hyde, R. (1954). The value of crafts in psychiatric occupational therapy. *American Journal of Occupational Therapy, 8,* 104-106.

Peloquin, S.M. (1991). Occupational therapy service: Individual and collective understandings of the founders, Part 2. *The American Journal of Occupational Therapy, 45,* 733-744.

Pianetti, C., Palacios, M. & Elliott, L. (1964). Significance of color. *American Journal of Occupational Therapy, 18,* 137-140.

Rocker, J.D. & Nelson, D.L. (1987). Affective responses to keeping and not keeping an activity product. *American Journal of Occupational Therapy, 41,* 152-157.

Rothaus, P., Hanson, P. & Cleveland, S. (1966). Art and group dynamics. *American Journal of Occupational Therapy, 20,* 182-187.

Royeen, C.B., Cynkin, S., Robinson, A.M. (1990). Analyzing performance through activity. *AOTA Self Study Series: Assessing Function, No. 5.* Rockville, MD: American Occupational Therapy Association.

Scardina, V. (1981). From pegboards to integration. *American Journal of Occupational Therapy, 35,* 581-588.

Shing-Ru Shih, L., Nelson, D.L. & Duncombe, L.W. (1984). Mood and affect following success and failure in two cultural groups. *Occupational Therapy Journal of Research, 4,* 213-230.

Shontz, F.C. (1959). Evaluation of psychological effects. *American Journal of Physical Medicine, 38,* 138-142.

Slade, S., Falkowski, W., Muwonge, A.K. & Slade, P. (1975). Immediate psychological effects of various occupational therapy activities on psychiatric patients: A pilot study. *The British Journal of Occupational Therapy, 38,* 172-173.

Smith, P.A., Barrows, H.S. & Whitney, J.N. (1959). Psychological attributes of occupational therapy crafts. *American Journal of Occupational Therapy, 13,* 16-21, 25-26.

Steffan, J.A. & Nelson, D.L. (1987). The effects of tool scarcity on group climate and affective meaning within the context of a stenciling activity. *American Journal of Occupational Therapy, 41,* 449-453.

Steinbeck, T.M. (1986). Purposeful activity and performance. *American Journal of Occupational Therapy, 40,* 529-534.

Taber, F., Baron, S. & Blackwell A. (1953). A study of a task directed and a free choice group. *American Journal of Occupational Therapy, 7,* 118-124.

Weston, D.L. (1960). Theraputic crafts. *American Journal of Occupational Therapy, 14,* 121-123.

Weston, D.L. (1961). The dimensions of crafts. *American Journal of Occupational Therapy, 15,* 1-5.

Williamson, G.G. (1982). The heritage of activity: Development of theory. *American Journal of Occupational Therapy, 36,* 716-722.

Yoder, R.M., Nelson, D.L. & Smith, D.A. (1989). Added-purpose versus rote exercise in female nursing home residents. *The American Journal of Occupational Therapy, 43,* 581-586.